Drug treatment in psychiatry

Social and Psychological Aspects of Medical Practice

Editor: Trevor Silverstone

Forthcoming in this series:
Malcolm Lader
The Psychophysiology of Mental Illness

Drug treatment in psychiatry

Trevor Silverstone, MA, DM, MRCP, FRCPsych, DPM
*Senior Lecturer in Psychological Medicine,
and Consultant Psychiatrist,
St Bartholomew's Hospital, London*

Paul Turner, MD, BSc, FRCP
*Professor of Clinical Pharmacology,
St Bartholomew's Hospital, London*

Routledge & Kegan Paul
London, Henley and Boston

First published in 1974
by Routledge & Kegan Paul Ltd
39 Store Street
London WC1E 7DD,
Broadway House, Newtown Road
Henley-on-Thames, Oxon RG9 1EN and
9 Park Street,
Boston, Mass. 02108, USA

Set in Monotype Imprint
and printed in Great Britain by
Billing and Sons Limited
Guildford, London and Worcester

ISBN 0 7100 7861 7 (C)
0 7100 7862 5 (P)

Contents

Figures and tables

Figures

Tables

Preface

This book was written to provide an introduction to pyscho-pharmacology for all those who are concerned in the management of psychiatric disorders, whether in the community or in hospital.

We have attempted to place drug therapy on a sound physiological and pharmacological basis wherever possible. To this end we begin each clinical section by reviewing what is known of the underlying physiological and biochemical factors in the condition under consideration; we then proceed to discuss the pharmacology of the various drugs used in its treatment before going on to outline a recommended course of treatment. At the end of the chapters on schizophrenia, affective disorders, anxiety and sleep a list of relevant drugs is given together with doses and, where appropriate, our comments.

The form of presentation which we have chosen has led to some repetition; we consider this a small price to pay for a comprehensive discussion of a particular clinical condition, or group of conditions, within a single chapter. Rather than giving detailed references within the text, at the end of each chapter we have recommended suitable sources of further information.

We express our gratitude to Professor Linford Rees and to Professor Sir Eric Scowen for providing us with the opportunities for pursuing our interests in the field of clinical psychopharmacology. We also thank Mrs Gail Frampton for all the secretarial assistance she has given us.

TS and PT

General principles Part I

Historical introduction I

A desire to take medicine is, perhaps, the great feature which distinguishes man from other animals.

William Osler, 1894

A drug, according to the World Health Organisation, is 'any substance which when taken into the living organism may modify one of its functions'. Psychotropic drugs are those which have, through their action on the brain, an effect on normal and abnormal psychological processes.

Perhaps the first such substance to be discovered, certainly the first to be referred to in Western literature, is alcohol: 'and Noah began to be a husbandman, and he planted a vineyard and he drank of the wine, and was drunken . . . .' In fact it is unlikely that there ever was a time when alcoholic beverages were not used; certainly the Egyptians drank freely of them and there is a picture dating from 1500 B.C. illustrating the unfortunate effects of drinking to excess. The word itself stems from the Arabic *al kihl* meaning essence, and *alcohol vini* referred to the essential or most subtle part of the wine.

Several other substances which are both used and abused in present-day society have almost as extended a lineage as has alcohol. Opium poppy seeds have been discovered in Stone Age settlements in Switzerland dating from at least 2000 B.C. Homer described the action of nepenthe, which most authorities believe to be synonymous with opium, as giving 'forgetfulness of evil'. There is even some suggestion that the secret of opium, probably coming from Egypt, was closely guarded by the élite and was given to certain chosen warriors (heroes) before such epic battles as Troy. The habit of taking opium spread throughout Europe and the East in spite of warnings against intemperate use; until de Quincey, in the early nineteenth century, vividly portrayed the agonies which could come from dependence on

3

it, most Englishmen regarded opium as but a simple family remedy.

Another drug which acts on the central nervous system, known to the ancients and still with us, is marihuana, the derivative of *Cannabis indica*. A Chinese emperor writing in 2200 B.C. referred to its euphoric properties and advised that its use should be restricted, as in his opinion it was little more than a 'liberator of sin'. Perhaps the most famous users of marihuana, or hashish, were the assassins (whose very name derived from the word hashish), a fanatical thirteenth-century Persian sect who, when intoxicated, would recklessly commit the most brutal murders.

On the other side of the world, in South America, the leaf of the coca tree containing cocaine, was until quite recently as widely taken by the indigenous peoples of the Andes as alcohol in our society. Unlike alcohol, which is a sedative, cocaine is a central stimulant and allowed the Incas and their descendants to work prodigiously without fatigue. Because of this property its use was encouraged by the Spanish mine-owners.

Even stranger are the effects of *peyotl*, the sacred cactus of Mexico. This contains mescaline, a potent hallucinogenic compound, which so distorts the processes of perception that brilliant dream-like visions may be experienced. More recently other hallucinogenic substances such as lysergic acid diethylamide (LSD) have enjoyed a certain vogue and have even been employed to some extent in psychiatric treatment, although with doubtful effect.

The drugs thus far considered have all been taken in the first instance to obtain a state of pleasurable relaxation or contentment; it was only much later that the isolation of the active principle of opium and morphine, in 1817, and of cocaine in 1885, allowed a medicinal application.

An ancient remedy from India, *Rauwolfia serpentina*, which has always been used therapeutically rather than socially, turned out to be of considerable theoretical and practical interest. Indian texts have for three thousand years recommended the root of this plant, which contains reserpine, in cases of psychiatric disturbance, a recommendation which was found in the 1950s to be soundly based, and reserpine was among the first of the newer 'tranquillising' drugs (see chapter 5).

In 1952, the same year as reserpine was formally introduced into modern psychiatry, Delay and Deniker described the dramatic effect of the wholly synthetic compound chlorpromazine (Largactil, Thorazine) in cases of schizophrenia, and in so doing may be said to have inaugurated the sub-specialty of psychopharmacology which has grown so rapidly in the past two decades. As with many other important therapeutic advances, the use of chlorpromazine was based on a chance observation. Promethazine, an antihistamine drug, was noted to exhibit sedative effects, and chlorpromazine, which is chemically related to promethazine (they are both phenothiazines), was synthesised in the hope of increasing this sedative action. However, it was found that its range of activity was much wider, and it was soon being prescribed for a variety of conditions, particularly schizophrenia and mania.

Shortly after the synthesis and clinical investigation of chlorpromazine another breakthrough came with the discovery of the monoamine oxidase inhibitors. As in the case of chlorpromazine, this also arose out of an unexpected clinical observation, namely that tuberculous patients being treated with iproniazid became rather more euphoric than might have been expected. As a result it was suggested that if iproniazid did have a real mood-elevating action, it might be related to its ability to inhibit the enzyme monoamine oxidase, and thereby affect brain amine concentrations (see chapter 2). If this were so it was further reasoned that such compounds might be of considerable therapeutic benefit in cases of depression. Although iproniazid itself was soon found to be too toxic for widespread application, a variety of other less toxic monoamine oxidase inhibitors have been synthesised, and the introduction of this class of drugs has greatly stimulated investigation into the biochemical basis of depression itself (see chapter 6).

As frequently happens, the discovery of one major new drug like chlorpromazine leads to a hurried search for other members of the same chemical class which, it is hoped, will prove more effective than the original compound. In the course of such a search, drugs bearing a superficial structural resemblance to the parent compound may be found to cause clinical effects quite different from those expected. Such was the case with imipramine (Tofranil), which was originally synthesised in the hope of producing an iminodibenzyl derivative related to chlorpromazine with an even stronger sedative action. On clinical trial imipramine had little sedative activity but did exhibit a marked antidepressant activity—a property which had not been forecast. Since then many

5

other drugs in the same group (the tricyclic antidepressants) have been introduced (see chapter 6).

The newer synthetic drugs thus far considered, the phenothiazines, the monoamine oxidase inhibitors and the tricyclic antidepressants, have all been directed mainly at the more severe forms of psychiatric illness, the psychoses. There remains, however, a great deal of minor psychological distress, mainly manifested as anxiety or the somatic accompaniments of anxiety, which accounts for a considerable proportion of the conditions presenting in general practice and internal medicine. Therefore any drug that can relieve such anxiety symptoms will obviously have a ready appeal. The barbiturates, the first of which, malonylurea (barbituric acid, named in honour of St Barbara), was synthesised in 1864, are still considered by some to be the most effective, and certainly the cheapest, antianxiety compounds. There is, however, a considerable danger of drug dependence developing (see chapter 9) and other anxiolytic drugs have recently been introduced which are claimed to be less addictive and less sedating. Among the first was meprobamate (Equanil, Miltown) which swept the USA in the 1950s. It has, however, been largely superseded by chlordiazepoxide (Librium) which, according to one authority, has been prescribed in the past five years to more patients throughout the world than any other single compound.

Since the 1950s when most of the drugs discussed were originally introduced, largely, as we have seen, due to chance, there has been a spate of new variants. There are currently available at least twenty-eight phenothiazine derivatives, nine tricyclic antidepressants, nine monoamine oxidase inhibitors, and twenty-five non-barbiturate sedatives and hypnotics. Not only the variety, but also the total number, of prescriptions for these drugs are rising rapidly.

Furthermore, it has become almost impossible to keep up with the enormous volume of published material pouring out each year. In 1969 the number of papers written on psychopharmacology alone was over 3,500 and the USA Government has considered it necessary to create a special department within its National Institute of Mental Health to cope with the monumental task of coding and indexing this flood of papers.

In a welcome attempt to provide some shape and order to this welter of information, and to assist the study of psychopharmacology generally, a committee of the World Health Organisation

6

has recently suggested the following classification of psychotropic drugs.

1 *Neuroleptics:* drugs with therapeutic effects on psychoses and other types of psychiatric disorder. In addition they usually produce extrapyramidal effects, such as tremor and rigidity.
(a) Phenothiazines: e.g. chlorpromazine (Largactil, Thorazine)
(b) Thioxanthenes: e.g. thiothixene (Navane)
(c) Butyrophenones: e.g. haloperidol (Serenace, Haldol)
(d) Diphenylbutylpiperidines: e.g. pimozide (Orap)
(e) Reserpine derivatives

2 *Anxiolytic sedatives:* substances that reduce pathological anxiety, tension and agitation, without therapeutic effect on disturbed cognitive or perceptual processes. These drugs usually raise the convulsive threshold and do not produce extrapyramidal or autonomic effects. They may produce drug dependence.
(a) Propanediols: e.g. meprobamate (Equanil, Miltown)
(b) Benzodiazepines: e.g. chlordiazepoxide (Librium)
(c) Barbiturates: e.g. amylobarbitone sodium (Sodium Amytal)

3 *Antidepressants:* drugs effective in the treatment of pathological depressive states.
(a) Monoamine oxidase inhibitors: e.g. phenelzine (Nardil)
(b) Tricyclic compounds: e.g. imipramine (Tofranil)

4 *Psychostimulants:* drugs that increase the level of alertness and/or motivation.
(a) Amphetamines: e.g. dexamphetamine (Dexedrine)
(b) Caffeine

5 *Psychodysleptics:* drugs producing abnormal mental phenomena, particularly in the cognitive and perceptual spheres.
(a) Lysergic acid diethylamide
(b) Mescaline
(c) Psylocybin
(d) Dimethyltryptophan
(e) Cannabis

The above classification will be used throughout this book. The compounds are discussed in association with the various conditions covered. Each chapter consists of an introduction to the underlying physiology and pathology of the given conditions (as far as it is known); this is followed by a discussion of the pharmacology of the

7

various drugs used in its treatment; in the final section a recommended therapeutic approach, using the drugs already discussed, is presented.

Suggestions for further reading

BAN, T., *Psychopharmacology*, Williams & Wilkins, Baltimore, 1969.

KALINOWSKY, L. B., and HIPPIUS, H., *Pharmacological, Convulsive and Other Somatic Treatments in Psychiatry*, Grune & Stratton, New York, 1969.

LEWIN, L., *Phantastica—Narcotic and Stimulating Drugs, their Use and Abuse*, Routledge & Kegan Paul, London, 1931 (reprinted 1964).

SHEPHERD, M., LADER, M., and RODNIGHT, R., *Clinical Psychopharmacology*, English Universities Press, London, 1968.

WORLD HEALTH ORGANISATION, *Research in Psychopharmacology*, WHO Technical Report, Series No. 371, 1967.

Pharmacology of central nervous system transmission

Neurohumoral transmission

The effects of drugs on mood, perception and consciousness can best be understood in terms of their actions on the underlying chemical mechanisms responsible for normal function of the central nervous system.

The contacts between one nerve cell and another within the central nervous system as well as in the peripheral autonomic ganglia are called 'synapses'. This term was first introduced by Sherrington in 1897 and is derived from the Greek word *synopsis*, meaning 'clasp'. It reflects the intimate nature of the contact between cells, which Sherrington, like others before him, recognised to be present.

The mechanism by which nerve impulses are propagated from one cell across the synapse to the other was a matter of considerable controversy until the middle of this century. According to one school of thought, synaptic transmission could be explained solely in terms of electrical events, whereas a second school of thought maintained that nerve impulses were transmitted by chemical substances released from the nerve endings. This idea was strengthened at the turn of the century by the observations of Lewandowsky and Langley that injection of extracts from adrenal glands produced similar effects in experimental animals to stimulation of sympathetic nerves. Elliott, in 1904, suggested that sympathetic nerve impulses released minute amounts of an adrenaline-like substance in close contact with the effector cells. In 1907, Dixon drew attention to the close similarity between the effects of the alkaloid muscarine and responses to vagal stimulation, and put forward the hypothesis that such stimulation liberated a muscarine-like substance, which acted as a chemical transmitter of the impulses to the effector cell. It was not until 1921, however, that Loewi demonstrated that stimulation of the vagus nerve of one frog heart released a substance into the perfusion fluid which slowed the rate of a second heart when the perfusion fluid flowed through it. Loewi and Navratil went on to show that this substance was acetylcholine.

It is now generally agreed that transmission at most, if not all, synapses in the mammalian central nervous system is mediated by chemical agents. These are released by action potentials which pass down the axon, and interact with receptors on the post-synaptic effector cell body to increase its permeability to ions and set up a further action potential within it.

Before a compound can be considered to be a neurochemical transmitter it should conform to the following criteria:

1 it must be present in the nerve endings
2 the neurone must contain the enzymes necessary for its manufacture and release
3 the presence of various precursors in the synthetic pathway should be demonstrable
4 there should be systems for the inactivation of the transmitter; where enzymes are involved, they should be demonstrable within the neurone or in its immediate vicinity
5 during nerve stimulation the substance should be detectable in extracellular fluid collected from the region of the activated synapses
6 when applied to the post-synaptic cell body the substance should mimic the action of the synaptically released transmitter
7 drugs which are thought to produce their effect by interaction within the transmitter should be shown to interact with it in the predicted manner under experimental conditions.

The last two criteria are probably the most important.

The bodies of nerve cells in the central nervous system are densely covered by synapses, and it is probable that they have more than one transmitter substance acting on their surfaces. It has been shown, for example, that at least three transmitters act on one type of cell, the Renshaw cell in the spinal cord, two of them being excitatory transmitters and one an inhibitory transmitter. Other experiments have shown that neurones in the cerebral cortex are inhibited by at least two distinct transmitter substances.

When it is recalled how difficult it was to demonstrate neuro-humoral transmission in relatively simple peripheral synapses, and that it is only in recent years that all the seven criteria listed above have been satisfied for them, the difficulties of unequivocally demonstrating transmitter substances in the central nervous system will be appreciated. In fact, the evidence for most of the substances which have been postulated to act in the central nervous system is only circumstantial and fulfils but a few of these criteria.

Among the numerous substances thus far suggested the most important are:

acetylcholine
noradrenaline
dopamine
5-hydroxytryptamine (serotonin)
histamine
l-glutamic acid
gamma-aminobutyric acid (GABA)
prostaglandins
substance P

Acetylcholine

Acetylcholine together with appropriate enzymes for its synthesis and degradation is present in the central nervous system. Histochemical studies have revealed probable cholinergic pathways to the cerebral cortex in the ascending reticular system and in the cerebellum. Microinjection techniques using iontophoresis have shown that neurones sensitive to acetylcholine are present in all regions of the central nervous system. In the spinal cord acetylcholine produces only excitation of neuronal activity, but in other parts of the central nervous system and brain both excitatory and inhibitory effects may be seen. The effects of acetylcholine in the spinal cord seem to be mainly nicotinic, while those in the cerebral cortex are predominantly muscarinic and can be blocked by antimuscarinic agents such as atropine and hyoscine. The central effects of these drugs differ, atropine having excitant and hyoscine depressant actions, and they probably depend on their anticholinergic effects on different groups of neurones in the brain.

Noradrenaline (norepinephrine)

Noradrenaline, unlike acetylcholine, is not widely distributed throughout the central nervous system, but is concentrated in the hypothalamus and brain stem. Fluorescent histochemical techniques have shown specific neuronal pathways which form and store noradrenaline; these are particularly localised in the hypothalamus. Such fibres fluoresce with an intense green colour. There is a marked similarity between noradrenaline-containing neurones in the brain and those in the peripheral sympathetic nervous system. In both, noradrenaline is highly concentrated in the nerve terminals with much lower concentrations in other parts of the cell and the terminal regions of both types of cell are similar, showing much branching and varicosity.

Microinjection techniques have demonstrated that noradrenaline has an inhibitory action on the Renshaw cells in the spinal cord, which are excited by acetylcholine. In the cerebral cortex it depresses neuronal activity, while in the brain stem both excitation and inhibition occur. Bradley and Wolstencroft found in experimental animals that about 80 per cent of the nerve cells in the medulla and pons responded to applications of noradrenaline, 20 per cent showing excitation and 60 per cent inhibition. Chlorpromazine, an adrenergic receptor blocking drug, appears to antagonise the transmitter actions of noradrenaline at those synapses where it is excitatory.

Dopamine

Dopamine is a precursor in the synthetic pathway of noradrenaline:

Phenylalanine ⟶ Tyrosine ⟶ Dopa ⟶ Dopamine ⟶ Noradrenaline

It is not surprising, therefore, that it should be present in the brain in about the same amount as noradrenaline. It does not have the same distribution, however, which may indicate that it has an independent action. Fluorescent studies have shown that dopamine is particularly localised in the caudate nucleus and neighbouring striatal areas, and its importance in this region has been emphasised by the demonstration that patients with Parkinson's disease have a reduced dopamine content of the basal ganglia. Drugs such as reserpine and alpha-methyl dopa which produce monoamine depletion in the brain, and hence reduce the dopamine content of the basal ganglia, produce clinical features of parkinsonism as an effect of over-dosage. Treatment of patients with Parkinson's disease with dopamine, administered either orally or intravenously, proved unsuccessful because dopamine does not pass readily from the circulation into the brain. However, its precursor l-dopa does pass into the brain, and is presumably converted into dopamine by the enzyme dopa decarboxylase present within the neurones. Wide clinical experience has confirmed its usefulness in controlling many of the features of Parkinson's disease, particularly the rigidity and difficulty in fine movement. However, l-dopa may itself produce a large number of undesirable central nervous effects including involuntary dyskinetic movements, sleep disturbance and a variety of psychological changes such as severe depression; agitation, confusion, delirium, paranoia, hallucinations, delusions and psychosis have also been reported. The extent to which such behavioural effects are due to dopamine acting itself as a central transmitter, or to its role as a precursor in the synthesis of noradrenaline, is at present not known.

It is probable that the effects of dopamine in the basal ganglia are opposed by acetylcholine and other muscarinic agents. One such compound, tremorine, produces a parkinsonian-like tremor in experimental animals which can be abolished by atropine and atropine-like drugs. The effectiveness of many established drugs in the treatment of Parkinson's disease such as benzhexol (Artane) and orphenadrine (Disipal) may, therefore, be due to their ability to block the central effects of acetylcholine.

5-hydroxytryptamine

Like noradrenaline, 5-hydroxytryptamine (5HT) is concentrated mainly in the hypothalamus and brain stem. Neurones containing this monoamine show a yellow fluorescence in contrast to the green fluorescence of noradrenaline containing neurones. Tryptaminergic neurones are thought to extend from the brain stem up into the cerebral cortex and hippocampal areas. Microinjection studies have shown no effects of 5HT on nerve cells within the spinal cord, but in the cortex and brain stem it has both excitant and inhibitory actions, like noradrenaline. Of the cortical neurones which respond to application of 5HT, about 30 per cent are excited and 50 per cent inhibited. In the medulla and pons about 90 per cent of neurones respond, 40 per cent being excited and 50 per cent inhibited.

The possibility that 5HT is a central transmitter was suggested by the finding that the potent psychotomimetic hallucinogenic drug d-lysergic acid diethylamide (LSD) is a potent inhibitor of

5HT in peripheral tissues. It was tempting to suppose that its central effects, too, were due to 5HT antagonism, but against this hypothesis was the observation that the derivative of LSD, 2 bromolysergic acid diethylamide (BOL 148), which is as potent a 5HT antagonist as LSD, was devoid of psychotomimetic effects. More recent evidence, however, suggesting that methysergide and cinanserin, both potent 5HT antagonists in peripheral tissues, may be effective in controlling manic psychotic states (see chapter 6) adds weight to the suggestion that 5HT may have an important role in central transmission. It is of interest that the excitatory effects of 5HT in microinjection studies could be antagonised by LSD, BOL 148 and methysergide, while antagonism of its inhibitory effects was rare.

Responses of cells to more than one transmitter

Bradley and his colleagues have studied with microinjection techniques the responses of cells in the brain and spinal cord to acetylcholine, noradrenaline and 5HT. In certain regions, such as the medulla, there were neurones which responded to all three substances; in some regions all the transmitters were excitatory, in others they were all inhibitory, and yet in others one compound might excite and the other two inhibit, or vice versa. In other regions of the brain more consistent patterns were observed, with all neurones responding in the same way to given transmitters, for example, acetylcholine and 5HT might have an excitatory action and noradrenaline might have an inhibitory action on all the neurones in the group. With such variations in response to the transmitter substances within the brain, it is not surprising that psychotropic drugs acting on these substances themselves show a wide diversity of effect.

Histamine

Histamine is present in the central nervous system together with its precursor histidine, in the same areas as noradrenaline and 5HT. Microinjection studies have shown that it depresses the excitatory threshold of many neurones in the spinal cord, and has both depressant and excitant effects on neurones in the cerebral cortex. Histidine, too, has a depressant action on cortical neurones.

Antihistamine drugs such as mepyramine and chlorcyclizine

antagonise both the excitant and depressant actions of histamine on cortical neurones, but they also antagonise the depressant effects of acetylcholine, noradrenaline and 5HT; thus the extent to which their central effects are due to antihistamine activity is uncertain.

L-glutamic acid

L-glutamic acid and related amino acids such as aspartic, cysteic and homocysteic acids have excitant effects on nerve cells in many parts of the central nervous system. They are widely distributed throughout the brain and are released from the cerebral cortex during states of cortical activity. Evidence for the role of l-glutamic acid as a transmitter at invertebrate neuromuscular junctions has been established, and it may ultimately prove to have an important role in the human central nervous system.

Gamma-aminobutyric acid

Gamma-aminobutyric acid (GABA) is an amino acid, related structurally to glycine and taurine, which is restricted in its distribution in the body to the central nervous system. Unlike glutamic acid with its excitatory neuronal effects, GABA depresses activity of neurones in the spinal cord and brain. Animal studies have shown that it is released from the cerebral cortex in quantities which vary with the level of cortical activity, and some pharmacologists have suggested that GABA is, in fact, the main inhibitory transmitter in the cerebral cortex. Caution must be exercised in such studies, however, to exclude the possibility that the amino acids are derived from cerebrospinal fluid or non-neuronal elements rather than from nerve cells. The place of GABA in central transmission is, therefore, still controversial.

Prostaglandins

Prostaglandin was the name given by Von Euler in 1935 to a lipid substance derived from human seminal fluid which contracted smooth muscle. Substances with similar pharmacological activity were found in the seminal fluid of sheep, and in extracts of prostate and vesicular glands. Today the term 'prostaglandins' no longer refers to a single substance but to a large family of closely related long-chain unsaturated fatty acids, all derivatives of prostanoic acid.

Several prostaglandins are present in the mammalian central nervous system, and are released from the cerebral cortex into a perfusing fluid when peripheral nerves are stimulated. This release is depressed by drugs such as pentobarbitone and chlorpromazine. Some of these compounds have been studied with microinjection techniques and have excitant and inhibitory actions on various neurones in the brain stem. Their action is prolonged when compared with other transmitter substances such as acetylcholine and noradrenaline, and, although their presence in the brain and release on nerve stimulation suggests some function relating to transmission, it may be that this is more concerned with control or modulation of transmitter release or neuronal excitability than actual transmission. It may be relevant to this hypothesis that some prostaglandins are released from phrenic nerve diaphragm preparations and from parasympathetic and sympathetic nerve endings during nerve stimulation, and it has been suggested that they may be part of a 'feedback' system regulating transmitter release or receptor responsiveness.

Substance P

This is a polypeptide which is found only in vertebrates and is localised especially in the phylogenetically oldest parts of the brain; levels are highest in the hypothalamus, thalamus, basal nuclei and in the dorsal columns and roots of the spinal cord. Although several studies have suggested either a transmitter action or a more general inhibitory effect, many of them were carried out with impure preparations. More recent experiments with purified substance P have yielded results in conflict with the earlier work; this may mean that most of the previously reported effects were due to impurities present in the preparations used, and should, therefore, be discounted.

Transmitter synthesis, release, uptake and metabolism

Although very little is known of the synthesis, release and metabolism of transmitters within the central nervous system, a considerable amount of information has been obtained in recent years about the handling of acetylcholine and noradrenaline at peripheral synapses, and it is probable that similar mechanisms apply centrally. For convenience, present knowledge regarding nor-adrenaline in sympathetic neurones will be discussed in more detail and, where appropriate, extrapolation from this to other transmitters such as acetylcholine, dopamine and 5HT, will be made.

Noradrenaline is present in sympathetic nerve terminals in several stores or pools, being localised in terminal ramifications of the neurone which have a beaded, varicose appearance. Adrenergic neurones in the brain have a similar appearance. Approximately 40 per cent of the noradrenaline is free in the cytoplasm and the other 60 per cent is in intro-granular stores, called 'synaptic vesicles', where it is bound to protein and hence is relatively resistant to metabolising enzymatic activity. Noradrenaline diffuses freely from the vesicles into the cytoplasm and from the cytoplasm through the cell membrane into the extracellular space. It is carried in the opposite direction by active transport mechanisms from the extracellular space to the cytoplasm, and from the cytoplasm into the vesicles. Binding of noradrenaline to protein within the vesicles probably represents a separate active process in which adenosine triphosphate (ATP) is involved.

There are two sources of the noradrenaline in the vesicles and cytoplasm:

1   Local synthesis from phenylalanine
2   Uptake from the extracellular space of noradrenaline which may either have been released locally, or have come from distant sites such as the adrenal medulla, or have been administered exogenously.

When isotopically labelled noradrenaline is injected intravenously into animals it rapidly disappears from the circulation. About half of it is metabolised, while the rest is actively taken up by adrenergic fibres and can be demonstrated radiographically in the cytoplasm and granules. When a post-ganglionic sympathetic nerve is cut and allowed to degenerate, its ability to accumulate exogenous noradrenaline disappears.

An understanding of noradrenaline uptake is important from the point of view of its inactivation after it has acted at the receptor site, for its binding within the cell represents a way in which it can be inactivated and used again.

The enzymatic metabolism of noradrenaline is largely dependent on two groups of enzymes: monoamine oxidase (MAO) and catechol-O-methyltransferase (COMT).

Monoamine oxidase is widely distributed throughout the body; within the brain it is present in larger quantities in the hypothalamus than elsewhere. It is concerned with the metabolism of a wide variety of compounds, including noradrenaline, dopamine and 5HT, and is located intracellularly in mitochondria at synaptic nerve endings, being partly responsible for regulating the cytoplasmic levels of these amines.

Catechol-O-methyltransferase is also widely distributed in brain tissue, and S-adenosylmethionine which is its cofactor is formed in the brain. Unlike MAO, it is responsible for the extracellular metabolism of noradrenaline which has diffused passively through the cell membrane or that which is released by nerve stimulation or drugs, and of catecholamines released from the adrenal medulla.

The steps in the metabolic degradation of noradrenaline, dopamine and 5HT are shown below:

It seems likely that when a nerve impulse arrives at the end of an adrenergic neurone, storage particles of bound noradrenaline, or synaptic vesicles, fuse with the neuronal cell membrane under the influence of calcium ions which enter the cell, and then discharge their contents into the 'synaptic cleft' or extracellular space. The released noradrenaline stimulates receptors on the effector cell surface, and is then either taken up again into the pre-synaptic neurone, or is metabolised outside the cell by COMT, or is carried away by extracellular fluid.

The series of events which have been described for noradrenaline probably apply to other transmitters. 5HT is synthesised within brain neurones from its precursor tryptophan and is metabolised by MAO. It is probably stored, and released in a similar manner to noradrenaline, and there appears to be a similar uptake process for this amine. Acetylcholine is synthesised from choline within brain neurones, and is rapidly destroyed on release by acetylcholinesterase. When acetylcholinesterase is inhibited there is some evidence of an uptake process for acetylcholine also.

Receptors

Neurohumoral agents and transmitters such as those which have been described earlier in this chapter are composed, like other drugs, of molecules. The result of their action on post-synaptic cells must eventually be explained in terms of an interaction of these molecules, or parts of them, with specific molecules on the post-synaptic cell membrane. The latter are called the 'specific receptors' for the transmitter or drug with respect to the particular effect. The term 'receptor' is usually limited to drug-cell or transmitter-cell combinations that indicate a sequence of specific effects. Other drug-cell or transmitter-cell interactions that do not initiate these specific effects, such as binding of drugs to plasma, binding of neurotransmitter to cell protein and to enzymes for transport, storage and biotransformation, are referred to in other terms such as 'secondary receptors', 'storage sites', or 'drug acceptors'.

Little is known of the chemistry of receptor substances in the central nervous system. It is possible to make certain tentative suggestions on their nature, however, on the basis of what is known about their counterparts in the peripheral autonomic system. Much of our knowledge of these has been gained from studies using specific receptor-blocking drugs, but often these drugs do not pass readily into the brain from the vascular system and so their usefulness in studying central receptors is limited.

Cholinergic receptors

The peripheral autonomic effects of acetylcholine are similar to those produced by the alkaloid muscarine and thus are known as its 'muscarinic actions', as distinct from its actions on ganglia and neuromuscular junctions which resemble those of nicotine, the so-called 'nicotinic' actions. Microinjection of acetylcholine into the brain and spinal cord, and studies in whole animals and isolated tissues with the tremor-producing compound oxotremorine, suggest that central cholinergic receptors are predominantly muscarinic and are blocked by compounds which block muscarinic receptors such as atropine and hyoscine. However, in several areas of the brain and spinal cord there is evidence of nicotinic receptors, or of receptors which appear to be intermediate between the nicotinic and muscarinic type.

Adrenergic receptors

In 1948, Ahlquist suggested that the effects of adrenaline at peripheral sympathetic sites could be divided into two groups with two types of receptor, alpha and beta. These were originally called 'excitatory' and 'inhibitory' receptors, respectively, because of their general tendency to produce excitation or inhibition when stimulated, but as there are important exceptions to this in both groups, it is better to refer to them only as alpha and beta receptors. Noradrenaline has predominantly alpha-adrenergic activity, the most important in man being vasoconstriction of arterioles in the skin and splanchnic area, producing a rise in systemic blood pressure, dilatation of the pupil and relaxation of the gut. The beta actions are mimicked by the synthetic sympathomimetic drug isoprenaline and include acceleration of the heart, dilatation of arterioles supplying skeletal muscles, bronchial relaxation and relaxation of the uterus. Drugs which selectively block alpha actions are known as adrenergic alpha receptor blocking drugs and include phenoxybenzamine, phentolamine, thymoxamine and tolazoline. The adrenergic beta receptor sites may be blocked selectively by a variety of related drugs including propranolol, oxprenolol, pindolol, alprenolol and sotalol. No sympathomimetic drug yet available has pure alpha or beta stimulating actions. When the alpha receptor effects of noradrenaline are blocked, for example by thymoxamine, its weaker beta receptor actions are seen, and even the potent beta receptor agonist compound, isoprenaline, can be shown to have weak alpha stimulating properties when its beta receptor actions are blocked with propranolol.

Although the alpha and beta receptor actions appear to be so different, it is probable that the actual receptor substance is the same, namely adenylcyclase. This enzyme catalyses the conversion of ATP to cyclic AMP, and is widely distributed in a large number of animal tissues.

Catecholamines, such as adrenaline, noradrenaline and iso-prenaline, have a central stimulating action, which gives rise to anxiety and restlessness; this stimulating action is probably due, at least in part, to stimulation of central receptors, through the same adenylcyclase-receptor mechanism as in the periphery.

Other receptors

Relatively little is known of the nature of the receptors in the central nervous system with which 5HT, dopamine and other transmitters might react. Indeed, there is controversy as to whether each transmitter has its own specific receptors, or whether the same receptor enzyme, or different parts of it, interacts with more than one transmitter. However, there seems to be good evidence that 5HT and dopamine, at least, have their own specific receptors in the central nervous system.

In the peripheral autonomic system it apears that there are at least two types of 5HT receptor, one of which is preferentially blocked by morphine (M receptor); the other is blocked by dibenzyline (phenoxybenzamine) (D receptor). Lysergic acid diethylamide (LSD) inhibits D receptor activity, but not M receptor activity. It is too early to be certain if central 5HT receptors correspond to one or both of these types, although there is some preliminary evidence that they are more likely to be D receptors.

Dopamine has some peripheral effects, for example on the renal arteries, which suggest that there are specific dopaminergic receptors and that it does not necessarily act through stimulating noradrenaline receptors. Animal experiments suggest that apomorphine, the potent emetic drug, stimulates similar dopamine receptors in the basal ganglia. It appears, therefore, that in some areas of the brain at least, dopamine produces its effect through specific receptors.

Microinjection and other techniques have suggested that most of the possible transmitter substances have both excitatory and inhibitory effects on different neurones. It has been difficult, therefore, to relate specific behavioural changes in animals or man to excessive or reduced activity of one or more transmitter substances. Recently, however, Dewhurst and Marley have put forward the hypothesis, based on experimental work in the immature chick, that cerebral amines may be divided into two functional groups. Excitant amines (Type A) have the general formula $R.CH_2.CH_2.NH_2$, where R is a fat-soluble planar hydrocarbon such as an indolyl or phenyl group. These amines, of which tryptamine is the most potent, produce behavioural and physiological excitation, and are presumed to act through specific Type A receptors. Depressant amines (Type C) are of general structure $R'.CH(OH)CH_2NH.CH_3$ where R' is water soluble, for example, catechol. Such amines, of which adrenaline is the most potent, produce all the phenomena of drowsiness or sleep, and are thought to act through Type C receptors. If this hypothesis is correct, then specific antagonists of Type A amines should reduce excitation and be effective in mania. Methysergide and cinanserin are potent 5HT antagonists and, in fact, have been claimed by some to be rapidly effective in controlling manic disorders. While these observations have added weight to the theory of Dewhurst and Marley, there are serious objections to it, the most important of which is that the central stimulant effect of amphetamine is reduced by measures which inhibit noradrenaline and dopamine synthesis, which is surprising if these compounds are sedative rather than excitant. Furthermore, catecholamines produce anxiety rather than sedation in man, and it is by no means certain that this is only of peripheral origin. Care must be taken therefore, in extrapolating from these experiments; it is a big jump from the immature chick to the adult human.

Figure 1 *Diagrammatic representation of a central monoaminergic synapse showing possible sites of drug action*
Right: A, granular pool of monoamine. B, cytoplasmic pool of monoamine. C, monoamine oxidase. T, precursors of monoamines (tyrosine, etc.)

(Modified from P. Turner and A. Richens, in *Clinical Pharmacology*, 1973, by kind permission of Churchill Livingstone.)

Mechanisms of the action of psychotropic drugs

From this brief review of the probable pharmacological basis of central nervous transmission, it is evident that a drug may interfere with central nervous function in a variety of ways (see Figure 1):

1 Inhibition of synthesis of transmitter substances
2 Production of 'false transmitter'

23

3 Increased precursor load
4 Depletion of transmitter from neurones
5 Inhibition of release of transmitter
6 Release of transmitter from neurones on to receptor
7 Monoamine oxidase inhibition
8 Uptake inhibition
9 Receptor stimulation
10 Receptor blockade

Inhibition of transmitter synthesis (site 1)

Several compounds are known to block the synthesis of one or more transmitters in animals, but little is known of their effects in man.

The synthesis of noradrenaline in man in inhibited by at least two substances which are used clinically. Alpha-methylparatyrosine inhibits the conversion of tyrosine to dopa by the enzyme tyrosine hydroxylase, which is the rate-limiting step in noradrenaline biosynthesis. This reduces tissue levels of noradrenaline, but 5HT levels remain unchanged. When used clinically in the management of patients with phaeochromocytoma, alpha-methylparatyrosine tends to produce sedation, while mild anxiety and insomnia often appear after sudden withdrawal of the drug.

Alpha-methyldopa is an antihypertensive agent which also reduces tissue levels of noradrenaline. This effect is due, in part, to inhibition of dopa decarboxylase, interfering with the conversion of dopa to dopamine. The enzyme is also concerned in the production of dopamine, histamine and 5HT, and levels of these transmitters in tissues such as the brain and heart are reduced at the same time as noradrenaline. Sedation occurs in almost all patients treated with methyldopa, but tends to disappear as treatment continues. When the drug is discontinued, a transient 'release-type' phenomenon of increased activity, excitability and insomnia may occur.

Production of false neurotransmitter (site 1)

A drug may be taken up into a nerve cell and metabolised so that it replaces the normal transmitter and is later released on nerve stimulation or by other drugs. The effects of such drugs on the receptors may either be similar to or different from those of the physiological transmitter substances.

The antihypertensive drug alpha-methyldopa already referred to in the previous section is thought to act in part by competing with dopa for decarboxylation by dopa decarboxylase so that the following biosynthesis occurs:

Alpha-methyldopa ⟶ Alpha-methyldopamine ⟶ Alpha-methylnoradrenaline

Alpha-methylnoradrenaline, therefore, replaces noradrenaline in equimolar concentrations in adrenergic neurones and may be released by nerve impulses as a false transmitter with noradrenaline (the physiological transmitter). Experimental evidence from animals and man on the relative activity of noradrenaline and alpha-methylnoradrenaline is inconsistent, but it seems unlikely that the central and antihypertensive effects of α-methyldopa can all be explained in terms of a false transmitter action of alpha-methylnoradrenaline.

There is considerable evidence that amphetamine, after releasing noradrenaline, is metabolised in nervous tissue to p-hydroxynorephedrine. This compound, which may then replace noradrenaline in adrenergic neurones, has less receptor stimulant activity than noradrenaline or alpha-methylnoradrenaline. The formation of p-hydroxynorephedrine with its lesser stimulant action may thus account in part for the tolerance which develops to the central and peripheral effects of amphetamine.

After inhibition of monoamine oxidase, endogenous tyramine, which is normally metabolised by this enzyme, accumulates in neural tissue together with its hydroxylated derivative octopamine. The latter accumulates in nerve endings in the brain, as well as peripherally, and is released by nerve stimulation to act as a false transmitter in competition with noradrenaline. The extent to which any of the behavioural changes, induced by monoamine oxidase inhibition, are due to the effects of octopamine is not yet known.

Increased precursor load (site 1)

Administration to an animal or man of a precursor of a neurotransmitter substance may lead to increased synthesis of the transmitter, provided that rate-limiting steps in the synthetic pathway are not already fully loaded. Thus, administration of l-dopa orally or parenterally leads to an increase of dopamine in the basal ganglia and of noradrenaline in some other tissues.

Tryptophan administered orally is hydroxylated to form 5-hydroxytryptophan which in turn is decarboxylated to 5-hydroxytryptamine.

$$\text{tryptophan} \xrightarrow[\text{hydroxylase}]{\text{tryptophan}} \text{5-hydroxytryptophan} \xrightarrow{\text{decarboxylase}} \text{5-hydroxytryptamine}$$

Similarly histidine is the precursor of histamine and is readily converted to it by the enzyme histidine decarboxylase.

Possible clinical implications of the use of some of these precursors will be described in later chapters.

Depletion of transmitter from neurones (site 2)

Reserpine is an alkaloid obtained from the roots of *Rauwolfia serpentina*, a climbing shrub indigenous to India and neighbouring countries. More than twenty alkaloids can be extracted from this plant with a wide variety of pharmacological actions, the most important of which is the depletion of tissue stores of catecholamine, dopamine, 5HT and histamine, particularly in the brain. This depletion probably involves inhibited binding of these monoamines in the intracytoplasmic granular stores so that they are more vulnerable to monoamine oxidase activity. The amine-depleting action results in two important therapeutic effects, namely the calming of manic and schizophrenic patients, and an antihypertensive effect in patients with hypertension. These therapeutic actions may easily become serious unwanted effects, however, for further amine depletion can itself produce severe depression (see chapter 6). Whether this is due to specific depletion of either noradrenaline or 5HT, or of both together, is not yet certain. Its dopamine-depleting effects result in parkinsonism which may be accompanied by choreoathetosis and cerebellar ataxia.

Alpha-methyldopa is another compound which produces depletion of noradrenaline, dopamine, 5HT and histamine from the brain. At least two mechanisms for this have already been described, namely inhibition of synthesis, and replacement of the physiological transmitter by a 'false' one. This depletion probably accounts for the sedation and depression which commonly occur with its use, and for the parkinsonism which may be seen with high doses over long periods of time.

The biosynthesis of 5HT in the brain is inhibited by p-chlorophenylalanine which blocks tryptophan hydroxylase activity, the rate-limiting enzyme for 5HT synthesis. Its behavioural effects are not marked, and administration of large doses to experimental animals does not appear to produce consistent stimulant or inhibiting effects. However, 'pre-treatment with p-chlorophenylalanine interferes with the characteristic pharmacological effects of other drugs, such as LSD, which interact with 5HT mechanisms in the brain. Its effects in man are not yet known.

Inhibition of release of transmitter (site 3)

Some antihypertensive drugs such as bretylium, bethanidine, debrisoquine and guanethidine are thought to interfere with peripheral sympathetic nerve activity by preventing release of noradrenaline from the nerve ending. They do not have significant behavioural effects in antihypertensive doses, possibly because of their failure to penetrate the brain. It is unlikely that any psychotropic drugs now in use act predominantly by this mechanism.

Release of transmitter from neurone on to receptor (site 3)

Sympathomimetic amines, which mimic the effects of sympathetic stimulation, may be broadly divided into two groups (see Table 1).

Table 1   *Classification of sympathomimetic amines into predominant direct and indirect activity*

Directly-acting	Adrenaline
	Noradrenaline
	Dopamine
	Isoprenaline
	Phenylephrine
	Methoxamine
Indirectly-acting	Amphetamine
	Ephedrine
	Hydroxyamphetamine
	Phenmetrazine
	Tyramine

The first group of catecholamines comprising adrenaline, noradrenaline, isoprenaline and dopamine, together with some other amines such as phenylephrine, depend mainly for their effects on direct stimulation of adrenergic receptors. The second group depend mainly for their effects on their ability to be taken up into the sympathetic nerve terminal and then to release noradrenaline from the synaptic vesicles in the nerve ending on to the receptor. They are, therefore, called 'indirectly acting' sympathomimetic compounds. This distribution is easily demonstrated in the peripheral autonomic system, for example in the eye, where depletion of noradrenaline by sympathectomy or drugs such as reserpine or high concentrations of guanethidine leads to abolition of the mydriatic effects of ephedrine, tyramine, amphetamine and phenmetrazine while the effects of phenylephrine and adrenaline persist.

It is probable that the central actions of amphetamine, phenmetrazine and other indirectly acting amines also depend on the liberation of noradrenaline and dopamine from central adrenergic and dopaminergic neurones. Animal experiments have shown that the central stimulant action of dexamphetamine is almost completely blocked by pre-treatment with reserpine, and by compounds which inhibit noradrenaline and dopamine synthesis. Its activity is restored, however, by very small doses of dopa which have no effects in the normal animal. The relative importance of dopamine and noradrenaline in mediating various components of the central effects of amphetamine is still not certain. The problem is complicated by the possible 'false transmitter' role of metabolites of amphetamine such as p-hydroxynorephedrine, already described.

It may well be that other centrally acting drugs act in part or whole by releasing one or more transmitter substances from central neurones.

Monoamine oxidase inhibition (site 4)

Inhibition of the action of the intracellular enzyme monoamine oxidase (MAO) leads to an accumulation within the nerve of monoamines such as noradrenaline, dopamine, 5HT and histamine. This occurs both peripherally and centrally. Monoamine oxidase is in fact a general term for a series of more specific enzymes which deal with the individual monoamines, but MAO inhibitors tend to inhibit the whole family of enzymes, and thus lead to an increase in all the amines. A large number of drugs inhibit MAO to a limited extent, including cocaine and amphetamine, but their main actions do not appear to depend on this property. In the case of other compounds, including the hydrazine derivatives iproniazid and phenelzine and the amphetamine derivative tranylcypromine, their pharmacological actions probably do depend on MAO inhibition. The hydrazine group produce a long-lasting inhibition by an irreversible, non-competitive inhibition of the enzyme *in vitro* and *in vivo*. In contrast, the harmala alkaloids, harmine and harmaline, produce a short-lasting, reversible competitive inhibition of the enzyme.

Inhibition of MAO enhances the elevation of brain catecholamine and 5HT concentrations and the central stimulation produced by precursors of these transmitters. They also reverse the central depression and amine-depleting effects of reserpine, and enhance the central stimulant effects of drugs such as amphetamine which release central stores of noradrenaline.

Uptake inhibition (site 5)

Uptake of noradrenaline into the adrenergic nerve terminals represents a major route of its inactivation, and it is probable that a similar mechanism operates with other transmitter substances including dopamine and 5HT. Inhibition of this uptake would lead to an increase in the activity of transmitter at the receptor site.

A large number of drugs have been shown to interfere with noradrenaline uptake, including many with actions on the central nervous system. Among these are the central stimulant compounds amphetamine and cocaine, the antidepressant drugs imipramine and tranylcypromine, and the tranquillising drugs chlorpromazine and reserpine. Because of the wide spectrum of clinical effects shown by drugs which possess this action it is probable that, in the case of most of these compounds, inhibition of uptake, though an interesting pharmacological phenomenon, does not contribute to the primary clinical effect. In the case of the dibenzazepine drugs, however, such as imipramine, it is probable that inhibition of uptake with increase of transmitter at the receptor site does account for its main therapeutic action. Furthermore, it has been suggested that at least part of the central action of the phenothiazine compounds, such as chlorpromazine, is the result of partial blockage of noradrenaline uptake at sites where the latter is acting as an inhibitory transmitter, so leading to a potentiation of its inhibiting effects.

It might be argued that facilitation of uptake with increase of intraneuronal breakdown of noradrenaline by MAO could lead to a decrease in the concentration of transmitter at central receptor sites. This, in fact, is one of the suggested modes of action for lithium salts in the prophylaxis of manic depressive psychosis (see chapter 6).

Receptor stimulation (site 6)

Some compounds may exert their central effects by a direct stimulation of central receptors. In animals apomorphine is thought to stimulate dopamine receptors, and the tremor-producing compound, oxotremorine may stimulate central cholinergic receptors. However, most compounds which reach the region of the receptor site appear to inhibit rather than stimulate receptor activity.

Receptor blockade (site 6)

Many drugs are known to block specifically adrenergic, cholinergic and 5HT receptors in the peripheral autonomic system, and it is probable that the central actions of some compounds are due to a similar mechanism. For example, the sedating effects of hyoscine may well be due to central cholinergic receptor blockade. It is probable also that phenothiazine drugs, such as chlorpromazine, owe the major part of their central effects to a dopamine receptor-blocking action, and the same may be true of the butyrophenones such as haloperidol. It is tempting to apply similar reasoning to the antihistamine compounds by suggesting that their central effects are due to histamine-receptor blockade in the brain. The therapeutic effects of 5HT antagonists in manic conditions have already been referred to, and these probably depend upon specific blockade of 5HT receptors.

It is evident that there are several different ways in which a compound may produce central nervous effects when considered in terms of its interactions with neuronal processes at the transmitter level. Many compounds may have several different actions. For example, chlorpromazine has been shown in different experimental procedures to influence the release of noradrenaline, to affect its uptake into the neurone, and to block dopaminergic receptors. It is difficult to be certain which, if any, is the most significant. Similarly, the MAO inhibitors have a marked effect on the uptake, as well as the breakdown, of noradrenaline, and it is uncertain on which of these two actions their central stimulant effects depend. Furthermore, the foregoing discussion has centred around the effects of drugs on the synthesis, release and uptake of transmitter substances and on receptor activity. It is important to remember, however, that drug actions also depend on other factors:

1 *Regional variations in the site of action* For example phenothiazines are thought to act primarily in the brain stem regions while barbiturates probably act in a more diffuse and non-specific manner through the cortex and subcortical structures.

2 *Membrane and intracellular processes* (other than those already discussed) Compounds may interfere with neuronal cell membrane activity and ion transport, so reducing the ability of the transmitter substance to trigger-off impulses in the post-synaptic cell. Other drugs may interfere with energy-releasing enzyme systems, so producing their effects beyond the receptor. Drugs which interfere with transmitter mechanisms may also affect these other, less well defined factors, and so their actual mode of action is even more difficult to define.

Suggestions for further reading

BARBEAU, A., and MCDOWELL, F. H., *L-Dopa and Parkinsonism*, F. A. Davis, Philadelphia, 1970.

BLACK, B., *Drugs and the Brain*, Johns Hopkins Press, Baltimore, 1969.

BRADLEY, P. B., 'The pharmacology of synapses in the central nervous system', *Recent Advances in Pharmacology*, J. M. Robson and R. S. Stacey (eds), Churchill, London, 1968.

COSTA, E., and GARATTINI, S., *International Symposium on Amphetamine and Related Compounds*, Raven Press, New York, 1970.

IVERSEN, L. L., *The Uptake and Storage of Noradrenaline in Sympathetic Nerves*, Cambridge University Press, 1967.

PHILLIS, J. W., *The Pharmacology of Synapses*, Pergamon Press, Oxford, 1970.

TURNER, P., *Clinical Aspects of Autonomic Pharmacology*, Heinemann, London, 1969.

3 Methods of studying behavioural effects of drugs

In most other areas of clinical pharmacology the therapeutic effects of a new drug may be predicted with some confidence on the basis of animal experiments alone. However, in psychopharmacology it is difficult to predict behavioural effects in man from findings obtained in animals. This is because:

1 there are few, if any, satisfactory animal models of abnormal human mental states such as schizophrenia, depression, mania or anxiety.
2 it is often impossible to be certain whether objective changes in animal behaviour after administration of a drug are due to sensory or motor effects, or both, or to changes in co-ordination, or even to hallucinatory effects.

In fact, it may not be possible to detect any therapeutic drug effect at all until the compound is given to patients suffering with a particular condition. For example, l-dopa has few, if any, central effects in normal subjects but can readily be seen to affect motor activity in patients with Parkinson's disease. Similarly, the antidepressant activity of the MAO inhibitors and dibenzazepine compounds can only be detected in patients with established depression. Although valuable clues may come from various animal tests, these tests often appear to bear little relation to clinical conditions in man.

In this chapter, tests will be briefly described which may be used to detect and evaluate central actions of drugs in animals and man, particularly those drugs to which reference will be made in later sections of the book.

Animal tests

There are a very large number of animal tests used to screen the effects of drugs on the central nervous system, and to study their mechanism of action. They can be classified in three main groups:

1 Pharmacological and biochemical
2 Behavioural
3 Electroneurophysiological

1 *Pharmacological and biochemical tests*

These include biochemical and histochemical studies of animal brain tissue to demonstrate localisation of possible transmitter substances and the influence of drugs upon them, as well as test procedures involving isotopically labelled drugs, such as auto-radiography (to show the distribution of a drug within various organs) and tracer studies (to determine the metabolic pathway of a drug).

A commonly used test for screening potential antidepressant compounds makes use of reserpine-induced hypothermia. Administration of reserpine to an animal reduces its body temperature, probably by monoamine depletion. MAO inhibitors and dibenzazopine derivatives, known to have antidepressant activity in man, reverse this hypothermic effect of reserpine. On the other hand, some other types of antidepressant drugs such as thiazesim do not possess this property.

2 *Behavioural tests*

There are a large number of tests in which the effects of drugs on animal behaviour may be observed. Many involve operant or classical conditioning procedures and may require a complex experimental design. One of the simplest behavioural tests is the Y maze in which an animal has to make a choice between the two limbs of the Y; the action of drugs on this choice can be measured and added effects of reward or punishment observed.

A rather more dramatic procedure is that measuring the 'muri-cidal activity' of cats, in which a mouse is released into a cage with a cat and the behaviour of the latter is observed.

Analgesic tests, of which there are a formidable number, may be considered to be behavioural, as it is now generally accepted that 'pain' represents a response of the whole organism to a noxi-ous stimulus (see chapter 13).

3 *Electroneurophysiological tests*

Neuronal activity within the brain and spinal cord is accompanied by changes in electrical potential across the cell membrane. The summation of these changes in large numbers of neurones may be recorded by superficial electrodes placed on the scalp, as in electro-encephalography, a technique widely used in human studies. In animals it is possible to implant electrodes in specific areas of the brain, or even localise them to individual cells, and so record electrical events more discretely.

A sophisticated modification of this principle involves introducing a minute amount of pharmacologically active substance in the vicinity of a neurone through a micropipette controlled by micromanipulators, and recording the potential changes produced with adjacent microelectrodes. Multichannel micropipettes have been developed by drawing out a number of glass tubes fixed together. The multichannel micropipette made in this way has closely adjacent openings at the common tip, the central channel of which may be used as a recording electrode, while the secondary pipettes can be used for the introduction of substances whose actions are to be tested. For recording extracellular potentials in the brain it is preferable to use electrodes with a tip diameter of 6μ or less.

As well as recording electrical changes in the brain and spinal cord, implanted electrodes may be used to stimulate discrete areas and study the effects of such stimulation on the animal's behaviour and physiology. The influence of drugs on such responses to electrical stimulation may then be investigated.

Tests in man

Sensory tests

1 *Smell and taste* Smell thresholds may be determined by delivering into the nose, through rubber or plastic catheters, metered doses of a test substance such as coffee or xylol. The number of doses necessary to produce a recognised sensation of smell of the test substance is taken to be the threshold dose. Taste thresholds may be measured by presenting series of substances in ascending concentrations to the tongue, the subject being asked to report what he tastes. These tests lack the sensitivity of tests of some other modalities, but when carried out under carefully controlled conditions, can reveal consistent changes in olfactory acuity

brought about by central-stimulant compounds such as amphetamine and phenmetrazine.

2 *Vision* A test of visual function which is mediated by the central nervous system, and is most useful in the monitoring of drug effects on the brain, is the critical flicker frequency (CFF). This may be defined as the fastest rate at which a flashing source of light appears to be flickering as opposed to being steady. It has a number of determinants including the luminance, wave-length, wave-form and light–dark ratio of the stimulating light; the area, portion and light-adapted state of the retina illuminated; the duration of exposure, and the size of the pupil. Age and constitutional factors may also influence the threshold and recently the importance of intersensory effects has been recognised.

By rigorously controlling these many variables in the experimental situation it has been possible to use the test for assessing the effects of central depressant and stimulant drugs. Alcohol produces a marked depression of CFF which is proportional to the alcohol concentration in blood and urine. Barbiturate drugs depress CFF and dose response effects may be obtained starting with doses as low as 50 mg amylobarbitone. Anxiolytic sedatives, such as meprobamate, chlordiazepoxide and diazepam, as well as phenothiazine drugs, lower CFF in doses which are too small to produce any subjective awareness of central depression.

Central stimulant drugs such as amphetamine and phenmetrazine increase CFF, as do hallucinogenic stimulant compounds such as psylocybin. Combinations of barbiturates and amphetamines in appropriate proportions may show mutual antagonism of effects on CFF. Thus, a mixture of dexamphetamine and amylobarbitone in the proportions found in Drinamyl produces no change in CFF when compared with placebo, although dexamphetamine alone produces a rise and amylobarbitone a fall in threshold. Measurement of CFF over a period of time allows a study of the duration of action of drugs and the influence of physiological variables on it. For example, the rate of excretion of amphetamine is markedly dependent on urinary pH, a low pH resulting in rapid elimination of the drug and an alkaline urine delaying its excretion. A comparison of the duration of action of amphetamine on CFF under conditions of urinary acidity and alkalinity showed that the magnitude and duration of elevation of CFF was significantly greater under alkaline than under acid conditions.

Drugs may also affect the peripheral components of vision such as extraocular motor balance, pupil and lens function and rod and cone activity involved in colour vision.

3 *Hearing* Just as the critical flicker frequency is a measure of a subject's ability to distinguish an intermittent light source, so the auditory flutter-fusion threshold (AFFT) is a measure of central auditory function. An interrupted random noise signal is used, and although the threshold varies greatly from subject to subject, it is very constant for any one person if measured, like the CFF, under strictly controlled conditions. Amylobarbitone 100 mg, diazepam 10 mg and chlorpromazine 25 mg and 50 mg significantly depress the AFFT, while amphetamine 10 mg raises it.

4 *Pain* There are a large variety of tests designed to measure pain thresholds in man, most of which are unsatisfactory and fail to show changes after administration of analgesic drugs in clinically effective doses.

Thermal stimuli have been applied, using hot and cold objects, but this method has many inherent variables such as the pressure of the warm or cold object and absorption of the heat by blood flow through the skin, which may itself be altered by the thermal stimulus. The use of radiant heat is also subject to this variation of local skin blood flow.

Electrical stimulation of the skin and tooth pulp has been widely used; it may discriminate between therapeutic doses of analgesics, such as aspirin and morphine, and identical placebos. There are large variations in threshold within subjects, however, and the skin and the pulp method may produce a hyper-irritable state which can persist for months. It is also possible to block dental pulp pain non-specifically, for example by adrenaline, which may confuse tests of centrally acting drugs.

The most predictable and sensitive methods of producing experimental pain involve causing muscle ischaemia with a tourniquet to occlude arterial flow in a limb, followed by exercise of that limb. The pain produced by this technique can be so intense that subjects may be very reluctant to repeat the tests on other occasions unless motivation is very high.

The intraperitoneal instillation of bradykinin to produce pain has been used in human volunteers, and has permitted determination of dose-response curves with non-narcotic and narcotic analgesic drugs, but its potential dangers are such that the method cannot be recommended for routine screening.

Tests of co-ordination and motor function

It is difficult to draw fine distinctions between sensory, motor and co-ordination tests in man, for even the sensory tests already described require a response from the subject which involves some co-ordination and motor activity. Nevertheless, in the tests previously described, the emphasis was mainly on sensory activity, whereas in the tests described in this section, attention is focused primarily on motor skills and on co-ordination of motor with sensory activity. It may not be easy to distinguish, however, between effects of drugs on local neuromuscular and spinal activity, and effects on the brain.

1 *Reaction time* This is the time taken for a subject to record a response to a given stimulus. In an alert subject this time may be very short, and electronic timing devices may be required to give a sufficiently accurate measurement. Even before the introduction of such equipment, however, it was possible to obtain results which showed effects of central depressant drugs. Almost a century ago Lauder Brunton used a system of pendulums and levers to demonstrate the effects of alcohol and other drugs on central function. It is customary to present the subject with a number of stimuli, both visual and auditory, in random order, and instruct him to respond to one particular stimulus by depression of a morse key or other form of electrical switch.

2 *Disc dotting* In this test of co-ordination, in which the McDougal–Schuster machine is most commonly used, a subject cancels, with a pencil, an irregular spiral of dots within circles as it rotates slowly on a turntable. Vision is restricted by covering the spiral with a lid in which there is only a small radial aperture. The cancellations begin at the origin of the spiral at the centre of the turntable and continue until the subject misses two consecutive target circles; the score comprises the number of 'dots' in the track up to the point where it has been broken.

A modification of this method consists of a rotating metal drum covered with an insulating layer in which holes have been cut in an irregular spiral course. The subject uses a steering-wheel to follow the course of holes with a lever and thus establishes electrical contact with them; the score is recorded on a digital counter. Drugs such as promethazine when given in single doses, have been shown to reduce performance significantly.

3 *Ball bearings* In this test of manual dexterity, the subject is required to pick up ball bearings (3 mm diameter) from a dish, using a pair of fine curved forceps, and then to drop the ball bearings, one at a time, into a small vertical glass tube with an internal diameter of about 4 mm. The score is the number successfully transferred to the tube in a given time.

4 *Tapping speed* This is a test of both co-ordination and motor ability, in which the subject taps on a morse key as rapidly as possible for a given period of time; a counter registers the number of contacts made.

5 *Hand steadiness* There are a variety of test situations designed to measure hand steadiness. Most require the subject to hold a metal rod or ring in close proximity to another metal object, such as a plate or wire, or to move one along the other, without allowing the two to touch. Contact of the metal objects completes an electrical circuit which can activate a bell, buzzer or light. The apparatus may be designed to give the subject a harmless but unpleasant shock when this happens.

6 *Pursuit rotor* In this test a point light source moves rapidly on a screen and the subject attempts to follow it with a rod at the end of which is a photoelectric cell. This records the amount of time for which the subject is able to keep the rod in contact with the light source and hence the accuracy of this movement.

7 *Reverse mirror drawing* This is a measure, not only of a subject's co-ordination, but also his sense of lateralisation. He sees the image of a design, such as a star, in a mirror in front of him, but the design itself is hidden by a screen. He is required to follow the outline of the design with a pencil held below the screen, controlling it from the mirror image. The time taken to complete the test, and the number of errors made, are recorded.

Psychological rating scales

Psychotropic drugs are usually prescribed for the relief of emotional distress or the amelioration of a disturbed mental state; two conditions which are very difficult to measure directly. To determine the relative efficacy of such drugs in these clinical situations we have to rely on a variety of rating scales, and other psychometric tests, a number of which are available. They fall into four broad categories:

1 Tests of intelligence and other cognitive functions
2 Scales designed to quantify overt behaviour
3 Ratings based on a standardised clinical interview
4 Self-rating scales completed by the patient himself

1 *Intelligence tests and other tests of cognitive function* These are perhaps the most familiar of all psychological measuring devices having been in use for over fifty years. Essentially, they attempt to quantify the ability of the subject to solve standardised problems and to learn new information. They are particularly useful in cases of suspected organic disease of the brain, and the most commonly used are the Wechsler Adult Intelligence Scale (WAIS), the progressive matrices, and the Mill Hill Vocabulary Test.

2 *Overt behaviour scales* These scales are among the earliest introduced for specifically psychiatric purposes. Among the first was the Phipps Psychiatric Clinic Behaviour Chart introduced in 1915 for nurses to use in making a daily numerical assessment of a variety of behaviours exhibited by their patients on the ward. A more recent example of this type of scale is in the Nurses' Observation For In-patient Evaluation (NOSIE).

The disadvantages of such measures are: first, they can be used only on hospital in-patients, and then only in a ward where the numbers and training of the nursing staff are adequate; and second, they afford very little information on subjective phenomena such as emotions, perceptions and beliefs.

3 *Clinical rating scales* These are basically designed to provide a quantitative estimate of the findings obtained during a clinical

39

interview. There are two types, each having a somewhat different aim:

(i) Scales designed to provide information over a wide range of possible symptoms; they are useful as an aid to diagnosis
(ii) Scales which are primarily intended for estimating change in individual symptoms occurring in specific psychiatric disorders.

While the second group of scales is only valid after a diagnosis has been made, it does allow more critical evaluation of drug changes within the particular given diagnostic grouping under study.

The complexity of rating scales of the first type ranges from the sixteen-item *Brief Psychiatric Rating Scale* to the '*Present Psychiatric State' Examination* covering over 400 items.

Of the scales designed to assess change occurring as a result of treatment within specific diagnostic groups, the most widely used include:

(i) *The Hamilton Anxiety Scale* in which twelve symptoms commonly associated with the diagnosis of anxiety state plus an impression of behaviour at interview are rated on a five-point scale (0= absent, 1 = mild, 2 = moderate, 3 = severe, 4 = very severe, grossly disabling).

(ii) *The Wing Scale for Schizophrenia* in which four attributes of schizophrenia, flatness and incongruity of affect, poverty of speech, incoherence of speech and coherent delusions are each rated on a similar five-point scale.

(iii) *The Hamilton Depression Scale* in which twenty-four features of depressive illness are separately considered and rated.

A variant of the specific diagnostic type of scale is the overall rating in which the clinical condition under study is rated as absent, mild, moderately severe, severe, extremely severe. In the global evaluation of drug treatment this is about as good as any of the more detailed scales considered above.

4 *Self-rating scales* With this type of scale, which does not require the presence of either a doctor, a psychologist or a nurse, the patient himself completes it by answering a series of multiple-choice questions. Here is a sample question from a self-rating scale used in the assessment of depression, the *Beck Depression Scale*

(only one of the following statements must be marked as reflecting the patient's feelings):

o I do not feel sad.
1 I feel blue and sad.
2a I am blue and sad all the time and I can't snap out of it.
2b I am so sad or unhappy that it is very painful.
3 I am so sad or unhappy that I can't stand it.

Another widely used self-rating scale for depression is the *Zung Scale*.

A number of self-rating scales for anxiety exist; the most widely used are the *Taylor Manifest Anxiety Scale* (TMA) and the *Institute of Personality and Ability Testing* (IPAT); however, a more recently developed scale, the *Morbid Anxiety Inventory* (MAI), appears to be more sensitive for measuring drug effects.

While such scales are obviously open to evasion or exaggeration by patients, in practice they are extremely useful and are economical of professional time.

The major difficulty encountered by patients completing such scales is the inability to decide upon one particular answer or category. (These scales are often referred to as *category scales*.) This is especially true of the Yes/No-type scales such as the *Eysenck Personality Inventory* (EPI) a very widely used measure intended to obtain an assessment of personality in terms of neuroticism, extraversion and introversion.

A recent innovation which avoids this difficulty is the *Analogue Scale* consisting of a straight line, usually 100 mm long, with one end labelled, for example, 'not at all anxious' and the other 'extremely anxious'. The labels can vary according to the condition or sensation being evaluated. Patients are asked to mark the line at the point which most appropriately reflects their state at the time. While there is considerable variation in the way different people use such a scale, it allows a very sensitive assessment of change occurring within a given person, and is particularly useful in monitoring drug effects.

Choice of rating scale

The choice of rating scale for any given project depends partly on the purpose for which it is to be used, and partly on the clinical condition to be studied. It is in most cases a compromise between exhaustiveness and exhaustion. If a great deal of information is required about a relatively small number of patients, and there are sufficient trained personnel to administer the scale, then the Present State Examination is without doubt the most comprehensive available instrument. However, most clinical studies of psychotropic drugs require relatively large numbers of patients and take place in clinics and hospitals where staff time is at a premium. Therefore for out-patient and general practice investigations the self-rating scales are probably the most useful. Their value is obviously much less in conditions such as severe depressive illness or schizophrenia where patient co-operation cannot be relied upon. It is particularly among these populations, usually in an in-patient setting, where the standardised clinical rating scales, like the Hamilton Anxiety and Depression Scales, and the Wing Scale for Schizophrenia apply.

Finally, it should be stressed that there is no intrinsic numerical value in the scores obtained by any of these scales; they merely enable a clinical impression or a subjective feeling state to be quantified. They do not actually measure anything directly.

Psychophysiological tests

Many psychiatric disorders are accompanied by physical manifestations. Centrally acting drugs may affect these manifestations, or may themselves have direct effects on various physiological activities. Only a brief review of some of the test procedures used in this field of psychophysiological measurement will be attempted here.

1   *Heart rate and blood pressure*   Heart rate and blood pressure may be abnormal in psychotic conditions, such as depression, mania and anxiety. Centrally acting drugs may also produce changes in these parameters, either through their central effect or through other peripheral actions which they possess.

In some circumstances it may be sufficient to record pulse rate by simply counting the radial pulse for a minute, and to measure blood pressure by the standard sphygmomanometer technique, after the subject has rested for at least five minutes. However, for a more accurate assessment of drugs on central and peripheral autonomic function, it is preferable to use electrical recording devices. While a standard electrocardiogram (ECG) will provide sufficient data to record heart rate, it does not provide the information in a useful way. By employing electronic circuits to perform the operations involved in heart beat recognition, counting and timing, by using a cardiotachometer, the need to count individual ECG complexes is avoided.

Automated recording of systolic and diastolic levels of blood pressure is more difficult, and in fact, there are few, if any, accurate methods which do not depend on arterial catheterisation, although systolic blood pressure alone may be recorded with rather simpler techniques. A commonly used method involves occlusion of the blood supply to a finger, using a small cuff. The point of occlusion is then determined by testing for a pulse distal to the cuff by means of: (i) a second cuff connected to a sensitive volume-displacement transducer, (ii) a small finger plethysmograph, (iii) a small crystal transducer strapped to the finger tip, (iv) by observing changes in optical density of the finger tip photoelectrically. Refinements of these methods permit continuous and automatic recording of systolic pressure.

2 *Skin resistance and skin potential* When a small electric current is passed between two points on the surface of the skin the resistance varies with the state of the subject's mental state. Measurements of the skin resistance levels are usually made over the palm; they often show slow and gradual changes as a function of the changing mental state of the individual; in the case of sleeping or drugged subjects the resistance may rise markedly, while the resistance falls rapidly following specific arousing stimuli.

Measurement of skin resistance changes are of considerable value in psychopharmacology, including the so-called psychogalvanic response (PGR) in which there is a change in resistance occurring as a result of a psychological stimulus. The technique is not simple, however, for the voltage and resistance involved is small, and requires sophisticated electronic recording apparatus and intimate electrode-skin contact to obtain accurate measurement. In addition, the stimuli used must be carefully controlled in order to keep arousal levels as constant as possible. Furthermore, it should be remembered that changes in skin resistance can occur with drugs which influence sweat gland function by a purely peripheral action.

3 *Plethysmography* Plethysmography consists of enclosing an organ in a rigid container called an oncometer and measuring the

volume changes of the enclosed part. This permits study of the nervous and chemical control of blood flow into the organ and changes in that blood flow induced by disease or drugs.

There are many different kinds of plethysmograph, but those used in psychopharmacology usually involve recording pulsatile variations in the volume of a finger or the forearm. Although these measurements of variations in organ volume are not direct estimations of rate of blood flow, under certain strictly controlled conditions, which usually involve sudden occlusion of the venous drainage, the pulse volume is a close index of the rate of blood flow.

Plethysmography is used particularly in studies of anxiety, mania and depression, in which physiological changes in blood flow can be demonstrated, and in the effects of drugs in these conditions.

4 *Electromyography* Tension of a muscle at rest can be a value able indicator of the mental state of a subject, particularly in conditions of stress and agitation. Although direct measurement of muscle tension in man is difficult, the electrical changes which accompany muscle activity can be recorded; it is also possible to record muscle tremor by suitable modification of the procedure. Electromyograms are usually obtained from surface electrodes placed over appropriate muscle groups but may be complicated by artefacts which make interpretation difficult. An alternative method is to use needle electrodes, but the major difficulty here is that only a very small volume of muscle tissue is sampled by the electrode tip and its precise localisation may not be easy to determine.

5 *Electroencephalography* A detailed discussion of the changes which can occur in the electroencephalogram (EEG) in mental and neurological disease, or in response to drugs, is beyond the scope of this book. Many physiological and metabolic variables influence the EEG and considerable experience is required to recognise changes which are due to extraneous factors. However, the EEG changes produced by certain groups of drugs are so consistent that their presence in a record can be considered as a strong indication that such drugs have been taken. Stopping drugs, particularly when the subject has become habituated to them, may also affect the EEG in important ways. For example, paroxysmal discharges may be seen in a significant proportion of subjects following barbiturate withdrawal, even in the absence of any previous history of epilepsy.

Because of the large number of variables which may modify the EEG, the following strictly controlled conditions are required for recording:

1 Complete routine EEG assessment, including sleep records, should be made on all supposedly normal subjects before admission to a study
2 All records should be taken by the same recordist
3 The same EEG apparatus should be used throughout
4 Subjects should be investigated at the same time of day and at the same time interval after the previous meal
5 Females should be investigated at the same stage of the menstrual cycle
6 Recording techniques should be standardised
7 Quantitative measurements based on short samples of the EEG should be made at a constant time interval after eye closure or eye opening

It is most convenient to use electronic methods of frequency analysis and summation to demonstrate changes in the EEG. A valuable additional technique measures 'evoked potentials', which are EEG responses evoked by specific stimuli such as visual or auditory signals. Many evoked potentials are of low amplitude and obscured by spontaneous background activity. However, as they are of a constant pattern, frequency analysis and summation procedures allow them to be picked out more clearly. The influence of drugs on these evoked potentials is of considerable interest.

6 *Pupillometry* Changes in pupil size are continuously taking place in association with alterations in mood and response to emotional stimuli. Arousal and fear produce pupillary dilatation while revulsion and disgust produce contraction. Centrally acting drugs, as well as drugs which modify peripheral autonomic activity, may also influence pupil size.

The pupil is supplied by both sympathetic and parasympathetic divisions of the autonomic nervous system and its diameter is readily measurable by photographic and other methods. Its responses to drugs, such as cholinergic and sympathomimetic substances, are consistent in repeated determination within subjects under standard conditions.

There are several methods available for measuring pupil responses. When rapid changes in diameter are being recorded, and when pupillary reactivity to light and dark are also being observed, infra-red pupillography is the most convenient. Infra-red light is reflected from the retina through the pupil, and is then monitored continuously on a recording apparatus, to show pupillary contraction and dilatation.

Where slower responses are being studied, however, this is often unnecessary and simpler photographic methods are equally acceptable; photographs of the eyes are taken and pupil diameter measured from the negatives after suitable magnification.

Among the centrally acting drugs which have been studied in this way, dibenzazepine derivatives such as imipramine produce pupil dilatation due, in part, if not completely, to reduced parasympathetic activity. Phenothiazines, butyrophenones and reserpine contract the pupil to varying extents. Pupillary response to locally instilled sympathomimetic amines may be influenced by centrally acting drugs, and this may provide valuable information on their basic pharmacological actions. For example, oral reserpine treatment reduces or may even abolish the mydriatic action of the indirectly acting amine ephedrine, amphetamine and tyramine while leaving the direct effects of phenylephrine unchanged. On the other hand, treatment with monoamine oxidase inhibitors potentiates the mydriatic actions of the indirectly acting amines.

Clinical trials

In psychiatric disease states, where there are virtually no appropriate animal models, potential therapeutic compounds can only be fully evaluated in patients. In addition, as there are so relatively few parameters in these conditions which can be measured accurately enough to assess the effects of drugs, and as the natural history may be unpredictable, it becomes difficult to relate change in clinical state to the effects of the treatment given.

For all these reasons it is important to design well-controlled clinical trials in order to evaluate the action of centrally acting drugs in psychiatry.

Clinical trials may broadly be divided into two types, the pilot trial and the controlled trial.

1   *Pilot clinical trial*   In this type of trial, which may include the first administration of a new drug to man, a relatively small number of subjects are studied in depth. The drug is first administered

in very small doses to normal subjects, or to patients, with informed consent having been obtained either from the subject or from responsible relatives. Test procedures such as those already described in this chapter are carried out before and at intervals after administration of the drug, together with toxicological studies, including haematology, liver and renal function, and electrocardiography. The toxicological tests are done at suitable times to show acute effects and to reveal any delayed hypersensitivity reactions which may occur. Metabolic and biochemical studies provide information on the absorption, excretion and biotransformation of the drug. Careful patient observation should permit a determination of the dose necessary to produce a desired clinical effect, if such an effect be present, together with the dose which produces undesirable effects; this allows the therapeutic ratio of the drug to be determined. At the same time possible mechanisms of action are explored.

The main object of this type of trial is to obtain some experience of the new compound, particularly with regard to its spectrum of activity and its toxic effects. This is done in an 'open' way, with both the investigator and experimental subject or patient aware of the nature of the investigation and the treatment used.

Having completed this part of the study, if the investigator feels that the evidence is suggestive of a useful therapeutic effect, the following two questions should be asked before proceeding further:

(i) Has the compound significant therapeutic effects when compared with an identical placebo preparation? (ii) Is the new treatment as good as, or superior to, the best treatment at present available? The answer to the first question will tell whether the drug is therapeutically active when investigator and subject bias have been exluded. Even if it were active, it would have little place in clinical practice if it were shown to be inferior to treatment already available. The controlled clinical trial is an experimental technique by which reliable answers to both these questions can be obtained.

2 *Controlled clinical trial* Bias on the part of the investigator or patient is a major source of error in the assessment of psychopharmacological agents. Many studies have shown that the greater the degree of control introduced into a trial of a new drug, and the

smaller the opportunity for bias, the less enthusiastic are the claims made for it; these findings are illustrated in Table 2.

Table 2 *Effect of research design on the outcome of clinical trials**

Research design	Studies reporting less than 70% patients improving no. %		Studies reporting 70% or more improving no. %	
No control groups or blind techniques	93	(42)	127	(58)
Control groups but no blind techniques	57	(54)	48	(46)
Control groups and blind techniques	66	(67)	32	(33)

* From *Psychopharmacology Bulletin*, March 1969

The most important measures taken to eliminate bias are (1) the double-blind technique (2) randomisation of treatments and (3) matching of patients.

1   *Double-blind technique*   The purpose of this technique is to ensure that neither investigator nor patient is aware of the treatment which the patient is receiving. For each treatment the new drug, a standard drug and an inactive placebo, are prepared in such a way that they appear identical. This may simply mean making tablets of the same colour, shape and size, but it may also involve flavouring to match the taste, and even introducing other substances to produce unrelated drug effects. For example, if a trial of a new dibenzazepine derivative is to be really double-blind, all the treatments used should produce some impairment of accommodation, dryness of mouth and interference with micturition and bowel function.

An important consideration when preparing a double-blind trial is to ensure that the formulation of the standard drug, which is usually a compound in current use, provides the same 'biological availability' as the generally used preparation. Otherwise, another error might be introduced, loading the result unfairly in favour of, or against, the new drug. 'Biological availability' refers to the ease with which the drug can be absorbed from the gastrointestinal tract; it can be influenced markedly by the excipient substances present in the tablet or capsule to provide bulk, even though they may lack significant pharmacological activity themselves, and may not appear to influence the cruder tests of tablet disintegration and dissolution.

2 *Randomisation of treatments* Having disguised the various treatments used in a study, it is important that the order of allocation be randomised.

Trials may be divided broadly into those (i) *within-subjects* and those (ii) *between-subjects*. In within-subject trials, all the patients receive each of the treatments being tested, and their responses to each treatment are compared to their responses to the other treatments. In between-subject investigations, each patient receives only one of the treatments under trial, and the mean responses of each group of patients receiving a particular treatment are compared to the mean responses of the other groups. Which type of trial is used depends primarily on the nature of the condition being treated. In a chronic condition, such as hypertension or rheumatoid arthritis, a within-patient study is suitable because patients may be expected to return to a similar base-line of disability when treatment is discontinued. However, in conditions which are self-limiting or cyclic in nature, such as the common cold, anxiety states or depression, this assumption cannot be made, and it is not reasonable to compare treatments within the same patient.

Randomisation of treatments is necessary in both within- and between-subjects types of trial. There are two important reasons for this:

(i) It avoids observer bias. If the investigator knows the order of administration of treatment, or that C regularly follows B which follows A, then the trial cannot be considered double-blind, even though the formulations used have been matched for factors such as colour, size and shape. Claims based on trials in which treatments with active drug and placebo were allocated alternatively, have not been substantiated when trials with true randomisation were undertaken.

(ii) It minimises 'carry-over' effects. The administration of one drug may influence the action of subsequent treatments in a variety of ways and so disguise their true effects. This is particularly important, of course, in within-subject trials. It is overcome by

49

using the 'latin square' type of randomisation. This is best explained by imagining that we have our three preparations, standard, new and placebo. Subjects are arranged in blocks of three, each of whom will have a first, second and third treatment. The latin square is so arranged that each preparation occurs once, and once only, as first, second or third treatment in any three patients, as shown:

A	B	C
B	C	A
C	A	B

It is evident that in the case of three treatments in three subjects more than one latin square is possible. For example the following is an alternative:

A	C	B
C	B	A
B	A	C

As the number of treatments and subjects increases, so the possible order of treatments increases, and the actual latin square used in any one study is decided by randomisation techniques which are best employed with the help of a statistician.

3 *Matching of patients* Among the factors that influence a patient's response to drugs are age, sex, duration and severity of the condition which is being treated. In order to obtain a valid comparison of the activities of various preparations, therefore, it is desirable to match patients within treatment groups for these various factors. This may prove impossible, however, particularly if the condition is relatively uncommon. As many factors as possible should be matched, and the limitations imposed by others which are unmatched should be recognised.

Under this heading may be mentioned variations in drug response due to differences in patients' weight. In animal experiments it is usual to give the dose of a drug on the basis of body weight, but in therapeutic practice in man this is seldom done except where toxicity is high, and dose-related. In fixed-dose studies blood and tissue levels of a drug tend to be higher in lighter subjects, and this may obviously produce differences in therapeutic response and toxicity. It may be wise, therefore, either to match patients for weight as well as the other factors mentioned, or to relate the dose to the patient's weight. In practice, however, these precautions are seldom taken, and this may account in part for the wide variations in response which are often reported in trials of centrally acting drugs. One way of monitoring such variations would be to determine the blood levels of the preparations used.

Statistical analyses

The final stage of a clinical trial is the statistical analysis of the data obtained. In the past many drugs have been introduced into clinical practice on the basis of unqualified clinical judgment on the part of a few investigators who had used the compounds in an open, uncontrolled way. The purpose of the measures already discussed was to eliminate observer and patient bias as far as possible, and the mathematical handling of the results obtained is the climax of this process. Table 3 shows the difference in enthusiasm for new drugs when statistical methods were used rather than conclusions based on the global judgments of patients or doctors.

Table 3 *Effect of statistical analysis on the outcome of clinical trials**

Basis of conclusions	Studies reporting less than 70% of patients improving		Studies reporting 70% or more of patients improving	
	no.	%	*no.*	%
Global judgment	175	(48)	191	(52)
Statistical tests	27	(59)	19	(41)

* From *Psychopharmacology Bulletin*, March 1969

Statistical methods require numerical values which can be analysed, and this is a major problem with psychotherapeutic agents. Whereas drugs such as diuretics and antihypertensive agents produce changes which can be quantified in terms of urine volume or blood pressure, anxiety and changes of mood cannot be evaluated in this way. The rating scales already described may go part of the way to resolving the problem, but they cannot be said to be entirely satisfactory, as the units used bear no constant mathematical relationship to one another. Nevertheless, where it is possible to obtain numerical values, as, for example, the number of subjects showing improvement, deterioration, or relapse, using an overall assessment, or in specific items on rating scales, then statistical techniques should be used. It is not the purpose of this book to describe them in detail, and readers are referred to specialist books on the subject, some of which are mentioned at the end of the chapter. Although simple tests such as Chi squared, Student's t and ranking methods may be sufficient where large and obvious differences between treatments are seen, more sophisticated methods are available which may show significant differences which are not so readily apparent. Particularly valuable are the multivariate techniques of analysis of variance, covariance and dispersion, which minimise differences in results due to other factors such as between-subject and between-time variations, so that the between-treatment differences may be more readily seen. Such methods of analysis are very complicated, however, particularly when several symptoms and signs are being assessed, and computer facilities are almost always essential for their use.

Where the results of treatment can only be assessed in terms of global judgment, as for example, whether a patient has improved or not improved, and where there are important ethical or other reasons for discontinuing the trial as soon as a statistically significant result is obtained, the *sequential trial* may be appropriate. This involves making preferences for one form of treatment against another, either within patients or between matched patients, and plotting these on a graph prepared from tables, once the statistical requirements for significance have been decided. When a line of significance is crossed, either for one drug against another, or for no difference between treatments, then the trial can be discontinued. For studies of centrally acting drugs, as for most types of clinical trial, a figure of 5 per cent is usually taken as being significant, so that the chances of obtaining a positive result when in fact it does not exist are less than 5 per cent; equally, the chances of not obtaining a positive result when one really exists are also less than 5 per cent.

Statistical techniques are complex, and wrong conclusions may be reached if an inappropriate one is chosen for a particular problem. For this reason, it is wise to include a statistician in the research team when preparing, prosecuting and analysing the results of a clinical trial.

Suggestions for further reading

AITKEN, R. C. B., and ZEALLEY, A. K., 'Measurement of moods', *British Journal of Hospital Medicine*, Vol. 4, pp. 215–24, 1970.

ARMITAGE, P., *Sequential Medical Trials*, Blackwell, Oxford, 1960.

ARMITAGE, P., *Statistical Methods in Medical Research*, Blackwell, Oxford, 1971.

HAMILTON, M., 'Drug therapy in psychiatry', *The Scientific Basis of Drug Therapy in Psychiatry*, J. Marks and C. M. P. Pare (eds), Pergamon Press, Oxford, 1965.

HARRIS, E. L., and FITZGERALD, J. D., *The Principle and Practice of Clinical Trials*, Livingstone, Edinburgh, 1970.

LADER, M., *The Psychophysiology of Mental Illness*, Routledge & Kegan Paul, London, 1975.

SALZMAN, C., KOCHANSKEY, G. E., and SHADER, R. I., 'Rating scales for geriatric psychopharmacology—a review', *Psychopharmacology Bulletin*, Vol. 8, pp. 3–50, 1972.

SMART, J. V., *Elements of Medical Statistics*, Staples Press, London, 1971.

VENABLES, P. H., and MARTIN, I., *Manual of Psycho-physiological Methods*, North Holland Publishing, Amsterdam, 1967.

4 Social and psychological aspects of drug taking and drug abuse

Drug costs and drug defaulting

The number and variety of pharmacological preparations for the relief of tension and the alleviation of disturbed behaviour has increased at a remarkable rate in recent years. In the United Kingdom during the period 1961–71 the number of prescriptions for psychotropic drugs rose from 32·2 million to 47·8 million per year, and it has been estimated that some 8 per cent of the adult population currently take some form of psychotropic medication each day at a cost of over £22 million. This accounts for at least 15 per cent of all prescriptions. In the United States it has been estimated that the proportion of psychotropic drugs to the total number of drugs prescribed is even higher (17 per cent) at an astronomical annual cost of over $700 million. It is, therefore, of paramount importance, in order to ensure that such a large slice of our resources is put to the best possible use, that psychotropic drugs are used only when they have been shown to be of proven clinical efficacy.

Furthermore, if an effective drug is prescribed in the informed opinion that it will ameliorate distressing symptoms, it is obviously equally important that the patient fully understands the directions for taking it, and takes it as directed. While this may seem a naïve truism, surveys have shown that many patients, particularly the elderly, have little idea of either the frequency or the number of tablets they should take, or for how long they should go on taking them.

It is not only the elderly who fail to take their medication as instructed; family doctors frequently come across numerous bottles of unused tablets in patients' homes. Among the most frequent excuses given by the patients for not taking their medication are: an improvement in the clinical state which leads to a belief that no further treatment is required; or conversely a

54

worsening in symptoms attributed, often rightly, to the tablets. There is therefore little point in prescribing large quantities of tablets if the patient is going to stop taking them as soon as an undesirable side-effect develops. This is particularly true in the area of psychotropic drugs, the great majority of which produce such effects.

Even without untoward side-effects, patients frequently default in their tablet-taking. In one psychiatric hospital out-patient study it was found, by assaying the drugs or their metabolites in urine, that *one-third* of the patients for whom psychotropic drugs had been prescribed, and who insisted they were taking them, were not taking any. Lest this might be thought to be due to vagaries peculiar to psychiatric patients, it should be pointed out that 50 per cent of patients with rheumatoid arthritis also failed to observe instructions, as did a high proportion of tuberculous patients on anti-tuberculous medication.

It appears that patients attending hospital are particularly liable either to misunderstand or ignore directions given. In general practice, however, advice is more closely followed, perhaps because of the closer doctor–patient relationship which exists.

Doctor–patient relationship

The doctor–patient relationship not only influences tablet taking but also has a profound effect on the outcome of any course of treatment. First of all, an understanding approach by the doctor will often be sufficient to relieve the patient of his symptoms, particularly where these are the result of worry or tension. In such a situation the benefit attributed to any medication prescribed may be due more to the doctor's manner, and his attitudes towards the drug in question, than to the pharmacological properties of the drug itself. This can lead to an overvaluation of the drug by the doctor and his patient. Even where a true pharmacological effect can be expected this effect may be modified considerably by the doctor–patient relationship. Not unexpectedly, doctors who evince a sceptical attitude towards the drug they are prescribing do not find such drugs nearly as effective as those who prescribe them with enthusiastic optimism. Patients can also influence drug response; any expectations a patient may have about the drug he is receiving can affect the outcome to treatment. Other factors also play a part: males seem to report fewer undesirable side-effects than females, and those of lower intelligence appear to do best overall when treated with psychotropic drugs. This latter finding may be related to the placebo effect.

Placebos

A good definition of what placebos are and how they are used has been formulated by Shapiro:

> A placebo is defined as any therapeutic procedure (or that component of a therapeutic procedure) which is given deliberately to have an effect, or which unknowingly has an effect on the patient's symptom, disease or syndrome, but which is objectively without specific activity for the condition treated. The placebo is also used to describe an adequate control in experimental studies. A placebo effect is defined as the changes produced by placebos.

Many authorities have remarked that this placebo effect was the basis of virtually all medication given before Withering used foxglove in dropsy; Sydenham found Cinchona bark effective in malaria; or Lind noted that fresh fruit was specific for scurvy. Eye of newt and leg of toad are, after all, unlikely to have much in the way of specific activity.

Recent critical interest in the placebo effect has been due in great measure to Beecher, an anaesthetist who observed that soldiers wounded in battle during the Second World War required analgesics less often (in 25 per cent of cases) than surgical patients with far less severe trauma, 80 per cent of whom requested analgesics. He found that a good many of these latter responded to placebo, but whether or not this occurred depended on a number of factors:

1 the nature and quantity of the placebo preparation given
2 the situation and manner in which it was prescribed
3 the social and psychological attributes of the recipient
4 the condition being treated.

1 *The nature and quantity of placebo* It has been suggested that the shape, size and colour of a tablet can each influence the placebo reaction. Very small tablets (which are by implication very potent) and very large tablets produce a greater effect than those of more moderate size.

Although normal subjects appear relatively unaffected by the colour of the tablet, psychiatric patients presenting with symptoms of anxiety or depression show a differential response to differently coloured pills. In one intriguing study, anxiety symptoms were found to respond most readily to green, whereas depression responded better to yellow tablets. Red tablets were the least effective in both conditions. As might be expcted, the greater number of tablets prescribed, the greater the effect within limits; for instance it has been demonstrated that while one 5 mg capsule of amphetamine was superior to a single identical placebo capsule in suppressing subjective hunger, three placebo capsules were better than one active amphetamine capsule.

2 *The situation and manner in which placebo is prescribed* The profound effect of the doctor–patient relationship in treatment has already been emphasised. Nowhere is this more marked than in placebo treatment. A study which illustrates this point well was carried out on patients presenting with gastrointestinal symptoms associated with diagnosed peptic ulcers. When patients were prescribed a placebo by a *doctor* who told them that they were getting a new medicine which would bring undoubted relief, 70 per cent of the patients reported definite symptomatic improvement; when prescribed a placebo by a *nurse* who informed them that they were receiving an experimental treatment of unknown efficacy, only 25 per cent benefited. Such variation in outcome in response to the status of the 'healer' and expectation of the patient is undoubtedly the reason why so many more of the seventeenth-century invalids in England preferred being 'touched' by King Charles II, to similar treatment from less exalted figures. It is estimated that this monarch touched over 90,000 patients during his nineteen-year reign.

3 *The social and psychological attributes of the recipient* Although the factors discussed above play a large part in determining the strength of the placebo effect some people appear more likely to react to placebo medication than others. As it would be clinically helpful if such placebo reactors (or responders) could be readily identified many attempts have been made to describe the characteristics which distinguish them from non-reactors. Unfortunately, the findings do not really allow of a clear-cut definition of the placebo reactor. Nevertheless, there appears to be general agreement

that the placebo reactor tends to be found more often among younger patients, particularly those of lower intelligence. There is no consistent sex difference, although some investigators have observed more frequent placebo responses in women. Most observers have remarked on the sociability and the apparent desire to please exhibited by the placebo reactor, and a relatively high level of anxiety has also been noted. Although perhaps more anxious in the treatment situation than non-reactors, the placebo reactors do not show widespread neurotic traits and are usually of a stable, rather outgoing personality. It is particularly important to recognise the corollary of this, namely that a patient who is demanding in seeking attention, or particularly complaining, is unlikely to be a placebo reactor, and is thus unlikely to respond to inert medication.

4 *Condition being treated* From studies on the effect of analgesics and placebos on post-operative pain Beecher and Lasagna concluded that placebos are most effective in acute severe stressful situations, being of considerable benefit in post-operative pain, with some 30 per cent of patients noting relief. They have also been shown to produce symptomatic relief in other acute conditions, including headache, motion sickness, coryza, angina and anxiety.

5 *Mode of action* If placebo acted purely by suggestion then hysterical conversion symptoms might be expected to improve rapidly, but this is one condition where they have proved relatively ineffective. Comparing the effects of repeated placebo administration to those of repeated aspirin administration in a large group of women in labour, Lasagna and his colleagues observed that the time course of efficacy was very similar in both aspirin and placebo; the placebo response was by no means 'all or none'. Similarly the placebo response may persist during the course of several weeks' medication whereas a suggestion response usually disappears within a few days.

Two observations which highlight the complex interaction between patient, the clinical staff and the treatment procedure are (1) morphine addicts, given saline injections instead of morphine, reported no withdrawal symptoms until the saline injections were stopped (2) the substitution of placebo for active medication, without either patients or ward staff being aware of the substitution, in a ward of chronic schizophrenic patients led to no deterioration in behaviour in the majority, and only 29 per cent relapsed; however, when the placebo was stopped and no tablets at all were given the relapse rate immediately increased to 85 per cent.

6 *Side-effects of placebo* In many placebo studies subjective reports of untoward effects often appear, with the following being the most frequent: *sleepiness, dryness of the mouth, headache* and *nausea*. It is obviously necessary to exclude placebo effects as a cause of such symptoms.

Often this may be difficult, as, for instance, when drowsiness follows administration of anxiolytic sedatives, or dryness of the mouth follows treatment with antidepressant drugs.

Occasionally, severe placebo reactions occur; widespread dermatitis, and angioneurotic oedema have been reported. Not only adverse reactions but true dependence to placebo have been noted on at least one occasion with the patient showing all the characteristics of the dependency state, including withdrawal symptoms.

7 *Use of placebo* A placebo may be given wittingly to a patient by a doctor in the hope that it might improve the patient's symptoms and in the knowledge that it is unlikely to make him worse. Few doctors appear to prescribe known inert substances in this manner nowadays, and with the increasing understanding of the psychological factors underlying many symptoms, the indications for such an approach are becoming fewer. It also raises ethical questions which were already being fervently debated at the beginning of the century. One physician went so far as to expostulate: 'Every placebo is a lie. Placebo giving is quackery.'

Much more frequently doctors prescribe medicines of doubtful efficacy, whose therapeutic effect is largely, if not entirely, dependent on a placebo response, in the mistaken belief that the drugs given have a definite specific pharmacological action. Although in many cases this belief is not very firmly held, the mere fact of prescribing relieves both patient and doctor—something is being done. It may be that in some ways we have not come far since 1906 when Cabot protested: 'We educate our patients and their friends to believe that every or almost every symptom and disease can be benefited by a drug. Some ignorant practitioners believe this.'

One survey of prescriptions in more recent times revealed that at least 20 per cent of drugs given to patients in the United Kingdom had no known pharmacological action.

Finally, the third mode in which placebos are employed is in experimental clinical trials (see chapter 3).

Drug dependence

Psychological and, in many instances, physiological dependence on drugs is an ever-increasing problem in our society, particularly among the young. Drug dependence is by no means limited to 'hard' drugs like heroin and cocaine, or to illegal drugs like cannabis. Numerically there is a much larger problem of dependence in commonly prescribed preparations containing stimulants of the amphetamine type, or anxiolytic sedatives such as barbiturates.

Furthermore, the frighteningly high prevalence of dependence on alcohol in many cultures (it is estimated to be 300,000 in the UK) swells the numbers of the drug dependant even more. This is without considering the dependence on nicotine and tobacco which is so widespread as to be considered almost normal.

Drug dependence has been recently redefined by the World Health Organisation as:

A state, psychic and sometimes also physical, resulting from the interaction between a living organism and a drug characterised by behavioural and other responses that always include a compulsion to take the drug on a continuous or periodic basis in order to experience its psychic effects and sometimes to avoid the discomfort of its absence. Tolerance may or may not be present. A person may be dependent on more than one drug.

Some further WHO definitions of the terms used are as follows:

Tolerance: 'the phenomenon of dose increase to maintain the drug effect'.
Physical dependence: 'an adaptive state that manifests itself by intense physical disturbances when the administration of the drug is suspended or when its action is affected by the administration of a specific antagonist'.
Psychic dependence: 'the intense craving and compulsive perpetuation of abuse to repeat the desired effect of a psychotropic drug'.

Drugs likely to lead to dependence all have in common the property of producing a rapid heightening of mood, or reduction of tension, followed by a feeling of 'let-down', which in turn can only be relieved by taking more of the drug.

Clinical features of dependence vary with the drug in question, and can best be considered individually in relation to the groups of compounds causing dependence, namely: (1) drugs of the morphine type (2) drugs of the barbiturate type (3) drugs of the amphetamine type (4) drugs of the cocaine type (5) drugs of the cannabis type (6) hallucinogenic drugs.

While the pattern of dependence may vary with the drug, the personality of the individual who becomes dependent tends to be similar. His personality can broadly be described as 'inadequate'; he is often someone who cannot cope with the normal frustrations of life without some form of psychological prop. Such a person usually requires immediate gratification, finding any delay intolerable, with a consequent tendency to impulsive and ill-considered behaviour. There are, of course, many people with similar characteristics who are not drug-dependent, but the addict has found or selected a particular way, namely the use of centrally acting drugs, of coping with his emotional problems and gratifying his psychological needs.

1 *Dependence on drugs of the morphine type* As was mentioned in the Introduction, the use and abuse of opiates dates from prehistory, but it was not considered a social problem until the eighteenth century. At that time the East India Company exploited the addictive properties of opium commercially, and this in turn led to the opium wars in the next century. Following the introduction of injectable morphine into military medicine during the American Civil War, a number of soldiers became dependent, a condition referred to at the time as the 'soldier's disease'. Heroin, originally produced as a non-addictive alternative to morphine, proved itself an even greater menace and most opiate addicts in Western society now take heroin, usually intravenously.

During the period up to the 1950s heroin dependence in the UK was largely confined to therapeutic addicts, i.e. patients who had originally been prescribed heroin or morphine for some medical condition. The remainder were doctors or nurses who had ready access to the drug.

More recently the pattern of heroin dependence has changed,

with far more young 'non-therapeutic' addicts being introduced to drug taking by their friends. The total number of heroin addicts in the UK is approximately 1,500 (just over twenty-five per million); in the USA the prevalence is over ten times as great with an estimated 56,000 heroin addicts (290 per million). In neither country is the problem quite so alarming as it is in Iran, where there are thought to be 50,000 opium addicts (6,550 per million) or Hong Kong with its 11,000 addicts (2,900 per million). Whereas in the USA the condition is largely confined to minority groups, this is not the case in the UK. Not only is the pattern and degree of addiction different in the two countries but the laws of each also show marked differences. Although heroin prescription in the UK is limited to authorised doctors working in drug-dependency clinics, addicts are allowed, and even encouraged to be treated on an out-patient basis obtaining strictly regulated supplies of heroin from their local pharmacist—in the USA it is illegal to prescribe heroin to addicts outside certain specified in-patient facilities under any circumstances, or for any individual to possess heroin. American addicts consequently resort to crime in order to obtain enough money to buy their supplies illegally and drug dependence has become inextricably bound up with criminality in the USA.

An addict's first experience of heroin is often during a weekend jaunt with friends, one of whom is already dependent and who encourages the other to inject himself. The first few injections may be subcutaneous but these soon give way to intravenous injections ('mainlining') which gives a more immediate sensation ('buzz'). At first, heroin injections will be limited to occasional weekend use, but self-injection soon becomes more frequent until, within a matter of months, the addict is no longer injecting heroin for positive pleasure; he is desperately trying to avoid the unpleasant effects accompanying withdrawal. These include shivering with pilo-erection (hence the term 'cold-turkey'), watering of the eyes and running nose, abdominal cramp followed by vomiting and diarrhoea. Individuals vary considerably in the intensity with which such symptoms are experienced (see chapter 9).

Perhaps the most disturbing aspect of heroin dependence is the high mortality of young, previously healthy, adults and adolescents. The mortality rate is twenty times that of non-addicts, and is due largely to secondary infection accompanying intravenous injections without sterile precautions, rather than to the direct action of the drug itself, although in some cases death follows an accidental overdose.

Treatment is aimed at withdrawal and abstinence, either gradually on an out-patient basis, or rapidly in an in-patient unit. Recent experience at the special drug-dependency clinics in the UK indicates that the former approach is likely to be more successful in the long term, particularly if accompanied by an accepting, supportive attitude on the part of all concerned.

2 *Dependence on drugs of the barbiturate type* This is probably the most widespread, but least-recognised form of drug dependence, apart from alcoholism. Some 80,000 people are overtly dependent on barbiturates in the UK (this is equivalent to over 0·2 per cent of the adult population) and ten times that number take a regular small amount of barbiturates; some twenty-five million prescriptions for barbiturates are issued each year.

Although reports of barbiturate dependence appeared in the 1920s the seriousness of the situation was not realised until relatively recently.

The great majority of cases were prescribed barbiturates as hypnotics either as part of hospital routine when they happened to be in-patients, or by their general practitioner. Cerebral activity is affected by even brief exposure to hypnotics. Cessation of the drug leads to a rebound disturbance of sleep with increased restlessness and dreaming, and the patient, trying to overcome these symptoms, reverts to the sleeping tablet he has been trying to do without.

Unlike other drugs of dependence, many more women than men are dependent on barbiturates. Increasing doses are required to offset tolerance and the characteristic picture of ataxia, nystagmus, dysarthria and drowsiness should alert one to the likelihood of barbiturate intoxication in a previously normal woman.

Serious withdrawal symptoms may occur after stopping barbiturates, particularly if the daily intake has been in excess of 1 g per day. These may include an episode of frank delirium punctuated by epileptic convulsions.

As with other drug dependency problems, withdrawal and subsequent abstinence are the therapeutic goals. In view of the serious nature of the withdrawal symptoms it is best carried out in hospital where gradual reduction of barbiturate intake can be attempted.

Doctors have a particular responsibility in preventing dependence on barbiturates. All patients prescribed these drugs should be warned of the risk of dependence. Requests for repeat prescriptions for hypnotics must be examined most carefully, and the common practice of routine distribution of night sedatives to every patient in a hospital ward should be reconsidered.

3 *Dependence on drugs of the amphetamine type* Soon after the introduction of amphetamine in the early 1930s its stimulant and euphoriant properties became widely recognised, and amphetamine abuse created clinical and social problems within a very short time. By the 1950s the contents of amphetamine inhalers were being extracted on a large scale and ingested by young people in the UK, Scandinavia, the USA, and Japan. When the availability of such inhalers was restricted, interest turned to amphetamine in tablet form, either alone or in combination with barbiturates (Drinamyl, 'Purple Hearts'). In recent years the use of injectable methylamphetamine (methedrine, 'speed') has become widespread. However, since its distribution in the UK was restricted to hospitals, there has been a gratifying reduction in its abuse.

Two quite distinct groups of people become dependent on amphetamine. First there are the otherwise relatively stable, often middle-aged women for whom amphetamine is prescribed to help them lose weight (see chapter 12); they seek repeated small doses of amphetamine to avoid the lethargy they experience when they are without the drug. The second group are much more emotionally unstable young adults or adolescents who take ever-increasing amounts to attain a state of euphoria and to ward off fatigue. As the effects wear off they experience a profound depression which can only be satisfactorily relieved by further amphetamine. Abuse in this group may lead to restlessness and irritability, resulting in unreasoning aggression towards others. On examination the pupils are dilated and there is a rapid pounding pulse. If amphetamine is taken over a long period a marked weight loss occurs.

Amphetamine psychosis can follow a number of large doses (50 to 100 mg) taken over a relatively short time. In this condition the patient is tormented by vivid auditory hallucinations and paranoid delusions. In some ways amphetamine psychosis resembles an acute schizophrenic episode but unlike schizophrenia the symptoms promptly wane when the drug is withheld.

As no physical dependence to amphetamine occurs, treatment is by simple withdrawal, although the possibility of a serious postdrug depressive state must be guarded against. Adequate social rehabilitation and psychological support will usually be required.

In the view of most medical authorities, amphetamines have little place in clinical practice, yet over four million prescriptions a year are still being issued for amphetamine and related compounds in the UK. Here again there would seem to be opportunity for the medical profession to take preventative measures.

4 *Dependence on drugs of the cocaine type* Cocainism, still a problem in South America, is becoming less prevalent in the developed countries where its use is largely confined to heroin addicts who take it to offset the sedative effects of heroin. Although heroin dependence remains as serious as ever most addicts, in the UK at least, no longer find it so necessary to add cocaine, and many drug-dependency centres are not prepared to prescribe it.

Cocaine, like amphetamine, is a central-nervous stimulant producing no physical dependence. When taken in large doses it leads to a state of over-activity and excitement, which may be accompanied by a most uncomfortable sensation in the skin reminiscent of insects crawling all over one's body (formication).

5 *Dependence on drugs of the cannabis type* Probably no drug is surrounded by more controversy and contention than cannabis, the mixture of substances obtained from the unfertilised flower heads of Indian hemp. There are at least four pharmacologically active substances in the resin: (i) tetrahydrocannabinol (THC) which depresses acetylcholine release within the intestine (ii) a second closely related substance (iii) a fat-soluble central-nervous depressant (iv) a water-soluble atropine-like substance. The taking of cannabis (marihuana, hashish, 'pot') is endemic in the Middle East, and, according to some, it so undermines the health and morals of the inhabitants as to ravage the community. In marked contrast to this view other authorities comment on the absence of any addictive properties, considering it a mild intoxicant significantly less harmful to society than alcohol.

Whether or not cannabis is less dangerous than alcohol must remain an open question. It is however a drug which acts on the central nervous system and as such is potentially addictive. Furthermore, the long-term dangers of cannabis have not been sufficiently studied for it to be pronounced free from harm; after all it was not until relatively recently that the long-term ill-effects of smoking were recognised. Until cannabis can be shown to possess positively useful qualities, the case for legalising it must remain weak.

The taking of cannabis has to some extent become confused with protest, since many adolescents take it as a gesture of defiance against what they consider to be the outmoded values of the Establishment. Most however remain only sporadic users and do not continue to take it when they themselves have family commitments. Fortunately very few graduate to taking 'hard' drugs like heroin. Nevertheless the danger of contagion remains; in an atmosphere where drug-taking is accepted, the progression from 'soft' to 'hard' drugs becomes that much easier.

The prevalence of cannabis smoking in the UK can only be guessed. One recent estimate put it at thirty regular users per 100,000. Its use is confined to young people, particularly university students who often take it in preference to alcohol. A sample of London University students revealed that 4 per cent could be described as confirmed users with a further 10 per cent admitting occasional use.

It is difficult to know exactly what the pharmacological effects are, as the subjective experiences vary so much with the social conditions under which it is taken. Regular users report a hazy glow of contentment, accompanied by a sharpening of perception and heightened sense of appreciation, particularly of jazz music (hence the prevalence of cannabis in jazz clubs); in contrast, naïve users often find that the effects, if any, are somewhat unpleasant. It produces little in the way of physiological effects apart from a rise in heart rate and a reddening of the conjunctiva. On psychological testing, cannabis was found to impair psychomotor performance in naïve smokers but not in regular users. This latter finding is surprising and has been advanced in support of legalising cannabis, the suggestion being that cannabis intoxication is likely to be less harmful when driving a car than alcohol intoxication.

High dosage can result in frank delirium and associated paranoid delusions followed by subsquent amnesia for the whole episode.

6 *Dependence on hallucinogenic drugs* We have already noted how preparations, like mescaline, with hallucinogenic properties can become incorporated into religious rites (see chapter 1). More

recently, particularly since the development of remarkably potent synthetic hallucinogens like lysergic acid diethylamide (LSD), the ingestion of hallucinogens has spread to other societies, partly in the belief that they may be therapeutic, and partly in the hope that the perceptual experiences produced will widen artistic horizons.

The amounts of LSD required to produce psychological effects are minuscule, as little as one millionth of a gram per kilogram body weight being sufficient, and of this, only one per cent actually crosses the blood brain barrier. Such small quantities can be readily disguised in sugar lumps or capsules and smuggling of LSD is consequently extremely difficult to detect.

LSD produces autonomic, sensory and emotional effects, in that sequence, over the course of some twelve to twenty-four hours. The autonomic effects include gastrointestinal activity leading to vomiting and diarrhoea, pupil dilation, pilo-erection and tremor. Following these there is a dramatic alteration of visual perception which allows the subject to perceive the world in a quite extra-ordinarily novel way. It is this distortion of perception which has so attracted to LSD certain intellectuals and artists who hoped to find a new stimulus to creativity through the drug. At the same time, or shortly afterwards, there is an awareness of a change in the quality of experience, which has been described in such terms as 'ecstatic', 'mystical', 'transcendental', but, as with many other drugs, these effects depend to a considerable degree on the social situation in which LSD is taken and the expectations of those taking it. Unfortunate sequelae to LSD can occur, particularly when the sensation of power and invulnerability displaces all caution. Under such conditions subjects may jump off buildings in the conviction that they cannot possibly come to harm. The LSD experience ('trip') may also give way to depression and consequent suicide.

The illicit use of LSD is confined to a few and the prevalence of regular users in the UK is probably less than one per 100,000. It is unlikely to have a useful place in psychiatric treatment.

Drugs and driving

All centrally acting drugs, if the dose is high enough, have a profound effect on motor skills and reaction time, as well as on the cerebral mechanisms underlying such functions as perception, anticipation and judgment of distance and speed. All these factors are obviously critical in driving where any impairment may well lead to a serious accident. In spite of the considerable potential risk attached to driving while taking psychotropic drugs, very little information is available on the subject. This is surprising in view of the ever-increasing number of centrally acting drugs prescribed and the equally expanding volume of traffic on the roads. Those surveys which have been done reveal an alarming lack of concern or even awareness of the problem on the part of most doctors and public authorities. A study in Wales showed that at least 3 per cent of all male drivers and 5 per cent of all female drivers were being prescribed drugs with a central action, the largest single group of drugs being the anxiolytic sedatives. The proportion of drivers being given drugs by doctors is probably even higher in urban areas. In a survey conducted in the UK by the Automobile Association 14 per cent of drivers admitted to having taken some medication in the previous twenty-four hours. Very few had even considered the possible effect such medication might have on their ability to drive, or had been warned by their doctors about it. In the United States some 11 to 16 per cent, and in Canada some 10 to 20 per cent of drivers take drugs regularly, of which at least a quarter are psychoactive.

Evidence of some association between the ingestion of drugs and road accidents has been obtained in California where 13 per cent of car-drivers involved in fatal single vehicle accidents (i.e. where only the driver of that car was to blame) had measurable quantities of drugs in their circulation. In most cases these were anxiolytic sedatives, neuroleptics and antihistamines, rather than drugs of abuse like cannabis or opiates. In Europe the number of drivers involved in road accidents found to have taken drugs, often in conjunction with alcohol, ranges from 10 per cent (Germany) to 16 per cent (Denmark).

Although such statistics provide sufficient cause for concern, there remains the possibility that some drivers, particularly the very anxious, actually drive better when taking moderate doses of anxiolytic sedatives. Unfortunately there is no evidence available on this point; the limited experimental work that has been done on the effects of anxiolytic sedatives on driving has been restricted to normal subjects. Furthermore, most investigations have been limited to measuring the effects of drugs on psychomotor tasks in the laboratory, or driving simulators; these can only provide pointers to the likely effects of drugs on driving, as they bear little relationship to actually driving a car in traffic, which is an extremely complex operation involving attention, perception, motor skills, motivation, and social attitudes. However there have been a few trials of drugs on driving a car in restricted traffic-free areas; the findings have been somewhat equivocal but, in general, there appears to be little impairment of car driving by experienced drivers after ingestion of therapeutic doses of anxiolytic sedatives. Alcohol, on the other hand, significantly impairs driving skills under these conditions.

Until more is known about the effects that centrally acting drugs have on the driving abilities of patients, the very least that every doctor should do is to warn his patients that their driving might be affected, and urge them to be ultra-cautious, even to the point of not driving, particularly during the first few days of medication, when the unwanted effects are most pronounced.

Suggestions for further reading

BALTER, M. B., and LEVINE, J., 'The nature and extent of psychotropic drug usage in the United States', *Psychopharmacology Bulletin*, Vol. 5, pp. 3–13, 1969.

BEECHER, H. K., 'Non-specific forces surrounding disease and the treatment of disease', *Journal of the American Medical Association*, Vol. 179, pp. 437–40, 1962.

DUNLOP, D., 'Abuse of drugs by the public and by doctors', *British Medical Bulletin*, Vol. 26, pp. 236–9, 1970.

FINCH, B., *Passport to Paradise*, Arco, London, 1959.

LEWIS, A., *Amphetamines, Barbiturates, LSD and Cannabis*, Department of Health & Social Security Publication No. 124, HMSO, London, 1970.

LOWINGER, P., and DOBIE, S., 'What makes the placebo work?' *Archives of General Psychiatry*, Vol. 20, pp. 84–8, 1969.

MILNER, G., *Drugs and Driving*, Kargen, Basel, 1972.

PORTER, A. M. W., 'Drug defaulting in General Practice',*British Medical Journal*, Vol. 1, pp. 218–22, 1969.

WORLD HEALTH ORGANISATION EXPERT COMMITTEE ON ADDICTION-PRODUCING DRUGS, WHO Technical Report Series, No. 273, 1969.

Clinical applications

Part II

Schizophrenia

5

Pathogenesis

Schizophrenia, which accounts for one-fifth of all patients currently residing in British hospitals, and for a similar proportion in many other countries, remains one of the least understood conditions in medical practice. In spite of years of painstaking research by teams of highly competent investigators in centres all over the world, almost nothing is known of its basic underlying pathology, or of its aetiology. There are three major obstacles to fundamental research in this area:

1 uncertainty of classification
2 inconsistency in diagnosis
3 inaccessibility of the living human brain to direct observation.

Schizophrenia may present in a number of ways; it is uncertain whether these are varieties of one illness, or several different illnesses, each with its own pathology and aetiology. Comparative studies have revealed that British psychiatrists in particular are more rigorous in making the diagnosis of schizophrenia than their American colleagues. This can lead to discrepancies when workers on one side of the Atlantic compare their findings with those on the other. Nevertheless, there is better agreement on the more florid cases, and certain schizophrenic patients are clearly recognisable as such whatever their cultural background. Probably the most significant barrier to advancement is the practical and ethical problem of examining the human brain directly. The biochemical and physiological changes within the depths of the brain, which probably underlie the strange and bewildering array of symptoms characteristic of this illness, remain largely inaccessible to direct examination. The majority of studies in this field have therefore been limited to the relatively crude approach of examining body

fluids, particularly blood and urine, in the hope of finding alterations in them which might afford a clue to pathogenesis.

Biochemical theories of schizophrenia

Although there is no certainty regarding the biochemical basis of
schizophrenia, a number of theories have been put forward.
Essentially they fall into two groups:

1 those which consider schizophrenia to be an auto-immune
disease with the basic disorder lying within the immunological
mechanism
2 those which consider that the fundamental biochemical disturbance lies within the central nervous system, resulting in the
production of an abnormal metabolite, possibly related to the
known hallucinogenic compounds.

These two groups of hypotheses are not necessarily mutually
exclusive but they emphasise different approaches to the problem.

1 *Immunological hypotheses*

(a) *Taraxein theory* According to Heath, the proponent of this
theory, there is a protein fraction (taraxein) which can be isolated
from the serum of schizophrenic patients and which produces
schizophrenic-like symptoms when given intravenously to non-
schizophrenic subjects. He believes that the primary disturbance
in schizophrenia lies within the septal area of the brain, and record-
ings made from the brains of schizophrenic patients in which
electrodes have been implanted apparently show specific abnormalities in the septal area. It appears that the active factor of taraxein
is in the gamma-G immunoglobulin fraction. Heath postulates
that this immunoglobulin factor, which he considers to be specific
to schizophrenia, acts as antibody to the septal region of the brain
producing an auto-immune reaction in that area.

Unfortunately for this hypothesis, other investigators have failed
to induce schizophrenic symptoms in non-schizophrenic subjects
with serum fractions from schizophrenic subjects. Equally, there
are very few corroborative reports on septal abnormalities in
schizophrenia, perhaps because the great majority of psychiatric
investigators are reluctant to implant electrodes into human brains.

Thus the taraxein theory remains largely unsupported by independent evidence.

(b) *B-lipoprotein theory*   Russian investigators have claimed that serum from schizophrenic patients has a more destructive effect on chicken red blood corpuscles than serum from normal subjects. They have also reported that schizophrenic serum inhibits the mitotic activity of cells in tissue culture and that sera from patients suffering from chronic schizophrenia show greater antimitotic activity than sera from patients with recurrent acute episodes. Attempts to isolate the particular fraction in the blood responsible for these phenomena yielded a β-lipoprotein, which possibly leaked out from cells as a result of a membrane defect in schizophrenics, secondary to an auto-immune response. When lymphocytes from schizophrenic patients were brought into contact with cultures of human nervous tissue destruction of the tissue culture cells and of the lymphocytes occurred. On the basis of their results the Russian workers suggested that in schizophrenic patients the proteins of the nervous tissue sensitise lymphocytes to produce antibodies which then react against other cells in the central nervous system. Such antibodies are not, however, necessarily restricted to schizophrenic patients as they could be found in the blood of normal subjects exposed to severe psychological stress.

Other workers have also reported the presence of abnormal lymphocytes in the blood of schizophrenic patients but the significance of such findings, apart from suggesting a possible auto-immune mechanism has not been established. These suggestions must remain very tentative at present, based as they are on studies of peripheral fluids and the membranes of isolated çells.

(c) *A-2-globulin theory*   Gottleib and his colleagues also observed that sera from schizophrenic patients altered the metabolisms of chicken red blood corpuscles. Detailed fractionation of this serum yielded a α-2-globulin which possessed the specific activity. Work from other centres has indicated that the α-2-globulin level rises with stress, and as with the Russian β-lipoprotein, it can be found in the sera of normal subjects as well. How this substance actually arises and what its biological functions are remains to be discovered, as does its significance in schizophrenia.

2 *Abnormal metabolite hypotheses*

(a) *Catecholamine metabolites* The metabolic pathways of the catecholamines within the central nervous system have already been reviewed (see chapter 2). It was suggested by Smythies that in schizophrenia there is a distortion of normal metabolism so that an abnormal metabolite with hallucinogenic properties is formed. At one time this presumed substance was thought to be adrenochrome (adrenolutin) formed by the auto-oxidation of adrenaline (epinephrine), and considered to possess hallucinogenic properties. Considerable doubt was subsequently cast on the presence of adrenochrome in human tissue as well as on its hallucinogenic properties.

Later workers imputed a fault in transmethylation of catecholamines as being of importance in schizophrenia, having noted that a number of hallucinogenic compounds were methylated. These ideas were given some support by the reported finding of 3,4-dimethoxyphenylethylamine (DMPE) in the urine of a high proportion of schizophrenic patients compared to its absence from the urine of normal subjects. DMPE shows up as a pink spot on a paper chromatogram and has given rise to the celebrated 'pink spot' hypothesis. More recent work has revealed that the pink spot is made up of a number of metabolites, many of which are present in the urine of normal subjects, although others appear to be restricted to schizophrenic patients. DMPE itself is apparently far less important than was at first assumed, and when administered to human subjects does not produce any schizophrenic symptoms.

Other findings also suggest a possible involvement of the catecholamines in the pathogenesis of schizophrenia, such as the exacerbation of symptoms of schizophrenia by methyl donor compounds, like methionine, particularly when administered with monoamine oxidase inhibitors. Arising out of this work, and of some potential clinical interest are two further unconfirmed reports: (i) That nicotinic acid (a methyl acceptor) may alleviate schizophrenic symptoms (unfortunately more vigorous testing has failed to find any therapeutic effect of nicotinic acid); (ii) That penicillamine, a copper-chelating agent, improves schizophrenic symptoms. This latter finding is thought to depend on penicillamine removing the copper ions necessary for the transformation of dihydroxyphenylalanine (dopa) to melanin, and thereby reducing the formation of harmine (a hallucinogenic compound related to harmalan).

More recently Kety has suggested that the biochemical lesion is an imbalance between dopamine and noradrenaline at certain synapses, as a consequence of a possible defect in dopamine hydroxylation. This hypothesis is based on two observations. First, amphetamine, which in high dosage produces a toxic psychosis closely resembling paranoid schizophrenia, has been shown to act on dopamine receptors within the brain. Second, effective neuroleptic drugs all appear to block dopaminergic pathways.

(b) *Indoleamine metabolites* Himwich and his associates noted that the concentration of tryptamine (an indole-amine derived from tryptophan) in the urine of schizophrenic patients rose during exacerbation of their illness and fell during remission. This observation, when taken with the findings that methionine plus MAOI produced worsening of symptoms in schizophrenic patients, suggested to Himwich that tryptophan and methionine may both be involved in the pathogenesis of schizophrenia. A possible mechanism would be the formation of N,N-dimethyltryptamine (known to be a potent hallucinogenic substance) from tryptamine, with methionine acting as the necessary donor of methyl groups. Attempts to examine the validity of this hypothesis by withholding methionine and tryptophan from the diet in the hope of alleviating symptoms, and supplementing the diet with methionine in the expectation of producing a worsening of symptoms, produced inconsistent results. It was only when methionine was given together with MAOI that any significant change in clinical state occurred. This particular finding however is just as much in favour of the catecholamine hypothesis as the indole-amine one. Reports that N,N-dimethyltryptamine is present in the urine of schizophrenic patients would, if confirmed, lend support to Himwich's hypothesis, but little information is available as to the specificity of this finding.

We would conclude from this review of current ideas that while there is as yet insufficient information for any one comprehensive theory explaining the pathogenesis of schizophrenia to be accepted with confidence, the catecholamine hypothesis, or a variant of it, seems the most promising at present.

Psychopathology

It is perhaps not surprising that no single theory of schizophrenia has obtained universal acceptance when one considers that there are a number of sub-types of the illness, and that its manifestations can vary considerably from patient to patient depending on the sub-type present, the cultural background and the pre-morbid personality. There are four main areas of psychological function which may be disturbed in schizophrenia, and correspondingly four varieties of the condition. The areas of malfunction involve perception, thought processes, emotional responsiveness, and motor activity.

Perceptual disorders

The most frequent of the perceptual disorders are auditory hallucinations (hearing voices). Patients can usually hear involved conversations between two or more voices (phonemes) which frequently make disparaging references to the patient, referring to him in the third person. Sometimes the voices will give the patient orders thereby producing unpredictable behaviour. Other hallucinations (i.e. perceptions without stimuli) can occur, such as sensations of electricity in the skin (tactile hallucinations) and strange smells or tastes (olfactory and gustatory hallucinations). Visual hallucinations are rare in schizophrenia, although characteristic of hallucinogenic drug-induced states. Auditory hallucinations also occur in chronic alcohol poisoning and acute amphetamine intoxication, implying a definite organic basis for their origin.

Thought disorder

Many schizophrenic patients, although not lacking in intelligence, are unable to put their thoughts together in a comprehensible fashion. This leads to a failure by the observer to grasp exactly what it is the patient is saying although the individual words and phrases appear to be quite normal. It is this peculiar lack of understandability of the train of thought which, when present, is pathognomonic of schizophrenia. Thought disorder of the schizophrenic type does not occur in any other mental illness and is not produced by any of the hallucinogenic drugs. Thus, hypotheses of schizophrenia based solely on a hallucinogenic drug model are unlikely to provide a complete answer to the problem of understanding the biochemical basis of the illness.

As well as having a disordered way of thinking (disorder of form), schizophrenic patients frequently believe quite irrationally that they are being persecuted, pursued or spied upon (paranoid delusions). Such delusions (or disorders of content) may exist without any disorder of form being present. Paranoid delusions, like auditory hallucinations, may also occur in amphetamine intoxication and in acute confusional states (see chapter 8). Other disorders of thought content include ideas that messages are being given to the patient on the radio or in the newspapers (ideas of reference) and the feeling that he is being controlled by an outside influence (passivity feelings).

Emotional disturbance

Characteristically, schizophrenic patients appear lacking in emotional responsiveness, presenting a blank, disinterested facial appearance (emotional 'flattening'); sometimes they may respond quite unexpectedly by laughing in the wrong places, or giggling to themselves (incongruity of affect); both these phenomena are particularly prevalent in the hebephrenic and simple forms of schizophrenia.

Motor behaviour

Certain patients gradually become less and less active, lapsing eventually into an apparently stuporous state (catatonia). This state may be interrupted by an outburst of violent activity (catatonic excitement) which ends as suddenly as it begins. Although extreme catatonia is now rare, less severe forms of inactivity and lack of drive are not uncommon.

Types of schizophrenia

Schizophrenia has been classified largely on the basis of the predominant symptoms or group of symptoms present. Whether or not the different types each have different aetiology and pathogenesis is not known.

1 *Paranoid schizophrenia* This is usually of acute onset and is the most common form in the elderly. Auditory hallucinations and

paranoid delusions dominate the clinical picture. This form is of good prognosis and the most responsive to neuroleptic drugs.

2 *Hebephrenic schizophrenia* This usually comes on gradually and is of less favourable prognosis. It is more common in adolescents and young adults. Incongruity of affect and schizophrenic thought disorder are the most prominent symptoms.

3 *Catatonic schizophrenia* This is the least common, usually having an acute onset in adolescence, and is characterised by catatonic motor symptoms (see above) with underlying thought disorder and delusions.

4 *Simple schizophrenia* This manifests as a gradual withdrawal from all social activity and a corresponding lack of motivation and drive. Flattening of affect is a feature, and thought disorder may be present.

Pharmacology of neuroleptic drugs

The drugs used in the treatment of schizophrenia were originally referred to as neuroleptics because of their ability to produce a state of 'neurolepsis' or calm indifference without loss of consciousness. They may be subdivided into several groups. These include rauwolfia alkaloids, phenothiazines, thioxanthenes, indole derivatives, butyrophenones and diphenylbutylpiperidines.

Rauwolfia alkaloids

Extracts of plants of the rauwolfia variety have been used in Asia for centuries for a number of conditions, including insanity and hypertension, but it was only some twenty years ago that the alkaloid reserpine was isolated and introduced into clinical medicine.

The calming effects of reserpine are probably related to its ability to deplete the brain of monoamine stores. Its therapeutic ratio is relatively narrow, however, and administration of higher doses may result in: mental depression which may be suicidal, extrapyramidal disorders with parkinsonism, choreoathetosis and ataxia (probably due to dopamine depletion in the basal ganglia), and finally to central respiratory depression and death. Diarrhoea, nasal stuffiness, fluid retention with cardiac failure and endcorine disorders, such as amenorrhoea, gynaecomastia and impairment of sexual function, can also occur. Increased gastric secretion can lead to reactivation of a peptic ulcer or to the development of new ulcers, possibly complicated by haemorrhage and perforation. In addition, the depletion of pressor substances resulting from reserpine administration may cause prolonged hypotension and bradycardia during the stress of anaesthesia and surgery.

Reserpine is readily absorbed from the gastrointestinal tract and from parenteral sites of injection. There are a variety of metabolites which are only slowly eliminated from the body. Reserpine appears to be taken up rapidly by lipid-containing tissues throughout the body, and is cumulative in action, so that any change in dosage should be carried out slowly and cautiously. It has been superseded almost entirely by the phenothiazines in the treatment of schizophrenia.

Phenothiazines

The discovery that the phenothiazine derivative promethazine possesses sedative and antihistamine actively encouraged the synthesis of other compounds in this group. Chlorpromazine, synthesised in 1950, was soon found to have pronounced calmative effects on disturbed psychotic patients. Since then it has come to be the standard compound against which other substances have been compared. Phenothiazines have a large number of pharmacological properties, and minor changes in their molecular structure may profoundly influence their therapeutic activity and the severity of unwanted effects, particularly the incidence of extrapyramidal reactions. All drugs in this group have in common the phenothiazine nucleus:

Derivatives are usually formed by substitution at positions R_1 and R_2. The side chains at R_1 may be classified into three groups: (i) dimethylaminopropyl (aliphatic) (ii) piperazine (iii) piperidine. The substitutions at R_2 include halogens, methoxy, acetyl, thiomethyl, and other organic radicals. Compounds such as promazine, which is unsubstituted at position R_2, are very much less active pharmacologically than derivatives with chloro- or trifluoromethyl substitutions at that position, such as chlorpromazine or trifluopromazine. It appears that the different substituents on the phenothiazine ring determine the site of action by altering the distribution of the drug, the more potent compounds having substituents which increase their lipid solubility and facilitate their transport into the brain. Their pharmacological actions depend on the electronic nature of the phenothiazine ring and involve electron donation in charge-transfer reactions.

1 *Antipsychotic and neuroleptic activity* This activity of the phenothiazines probably depends on their effects on brain monoamines, particularly dopamine. Animal studies have shown that they cause the accumulation of the O-methylated metabolites of noradrenaline and dopamine, and it is probable that they block central dopamine and noradrenaline receptors, causing a compensatory activation of dopaminergic and adrenergic neurones with an increase in transmitter release and extraneuronal breakdown. Phenothiazines also possess some peripheral adrenergic receptor blocking properties which may lead to orthostatic hypotension in the early days of treatment. In addition they have a relatively weak atropine-like anticholinergic action and weak to moderate anti-histamine and anti-5HT effects.

2 *Antiemetic activity* The phenothiazines are potent antiemetic drugs, preventing vomiting produced by other drugs such as apomorphine which stimulate the chemoreceptor trigger zone. An action on neighbouring medullary areas may be responsible for their usefulness in the control of persistent hiccough.

3 *Extrapyramidal effects* The therapeutic usefulness of the phenothiazines is to some degree limited by their extrapyramidal effects. Some authorities believe that their tranquillising potency correlates best with these effects when compared with their other adverse reactions; those phenothiazines with the strongest antipsychotic activity, such as trifluoperazine, also give rise to the highest incidence of tremor and abnormal movements. This would be expected if a similar biochemical mechanism of action, namely a blockade of central catecholamine activity, was responsible for both the therapeutic and toxic actions. More recently, however, it

has become clear that the association between the two effects (antipsychotic and extrapyramidal) is not essential for therapeutic efficacy. Drugs such as thioridazine possess antipsychotic effects equivalent to chlorpromazine but are less likely to produce parkinsonism. It may be that the phenothiazines act on two distinct dopamine-containing neural pathways; the antipsychotic effects reflect their action on a meso-limbic system and the extrapyramidal effects depend on their action within the nigro-striatal system.

There are four main types of extrapyramidal symptoms produced by neuroleptic drugs: (i) those which come on early in treatment and mimic the symptoms of Parkinson's disease (pseudo-parkinsonism) (ii) akathisia (iii) acute dyskinesia (iv) those which occur only after prolonged dosage and which are often exacerbated by stopping the drug (tardive dyskinesia). The pseudo-parkinsonism is thought to be due to a relative insufficiency of dopamine at the post-synaptic membrane (as in idiopathic Parkinson's disease) secondary to the dopaminergic blockade produced by the neuroleptic compounds; tardive dyskinesia on the other hand, is possibly the consequence of a compensatory hypersensitivity to dopamine which becomes more manifest when the dopamine blockade is lifted by stopping the drug. The symptoms of tardive dyskinesia are more choreiform in character and particularly involve the mouth and tongue.

4 *Other adverse effects:* (a) *abnormal pigmentation* Like the extrapyramidal effects of phenothiazine therapy, abnormal pigmentation is a dose-dependent phenomenon, but is only seen after long-term administration. Exposed areas of skin acquire a grey-blue pigmentation, and on histological examination the dermis is found to contain melanin deposits. Corneal and lenticular deposits in the eye can also occur and may lead to impairment of vision. Large doses of thioridazine over long periods may produce retinal pigmentation.

(b) *Jaundice* A cholestatic type of jaundice has been reported in up to 4 per cent of all phenothiazine-treated patients, although more recent surveys reveal a much lower incidence. The jaundice usually comes on within a few weeks of commencing treatment. It is not dose-dependent and appears to be a hypersensitivity reaction. Eosinophilic infiltration of the liver as well as blood eosinophilia accompanies the condition. Upper abdominal pain commonly

83

occurs, and the clinical picture may resemble cholecystitis or cholelithiasis.

Other uncommon hypersensitivity reactions include dermatitis and blood dyscrasias.

5 *Interactions with other drugs* Phenothiazines enhance the central depressant effects of many other drugs including barbiturates and alcohol. They also potentiate the analgesic effect of the narcotic analgesic drugs; this may be of therapeutic value in patients with severe pain, particularly where it results from neoplastic diseases and is accompanied by marked anxiety.

While they only possess a weak anticholinergic activity themselves, when combined with an anticholinergic compound prescribed to relieve parkinsonian side-effects, an atropine-type psychosis can occur due to the additive atropine-like activity.

6 *Absorption, fate and excretion* Phenothiazines are readily absorbed from the gastrointestinal tract and parenteral sites of administration, and are rapidly distributed throughout all the body tissues, the highest concentrations being in the lung, liver, adrenal gland and spleen. Within the brain there would appear to be selective distribution, highest concentrations being found in the hypothalamus, basal ganglia, thalamus and hippocampus. They are markedly cumulative, metabolic products, being detectable in the urine up to eighteen months after discontinuation of treatment in patients who have received one of these compounds for long periods of time.

Fluphenazine enanthate and decanoate are long-acting parenteral forms of fluphenazine which produce effective blood levels for up to twenty-one days and therefore only require administration once every two to three weeks. Severe extrapyramidal effects may occur during the first few days after injection.

Thioxanthenes

In these compounds the nitrogen in the central ring of the phenothiazine is replaced by carbon. The analogues thus formed appear to be no more effective than their phenothiazine progenitors.

Butyrophenones

Although the butyrophenone compounds are structurally distinct from the phenothiazines they share many of their pharmacological properties. Like the phenothiazines they cause accumulation of O-methylated metabolites of dopamine and noradrenaline within the brain, suggesting that they also block dopamine and noradrenaline receptors, thus causing compensatory activity of central neurones with monoamine transmitter release. In the peripheral autonomic nervous system butyrophenones such as haloperidol and trifluperidol selectively block dopamine receptors in the renal and mesenteric vascular beds, and it may be that a similar selectivity of action occurs in the central nervous system.

The butyrophenones are also potent antiemetic drugs, suppressing activity of the chemoreceptor trigger zone, and they produce extrapyramidal disorders similar to those accompanying phenothiazine medication. They also potentiate the sedative effects of alcohol, analgesics, anaesthetics and barbiturate drugs, and transient orthostatic hypotension can occur, due to peripheral adrenergic receptor blockade.

Diphenylbutylpiperidines

These compounds, derived from the butyrophenones, have a more prolonged duration of action.

Other drugs

Tetrabenazine This is a synthetic benzoquinolizine which retains some of the structural features of reserpine and has an identical pharmacology. It depletes the brain of its monoamine stores and this is probably the basis of its sedative and antipsychotic effects. Mental depression and extrapyramidal reactions commonly occur. Its dopamine depleting property is said to be useful in the management of tardive dyskinesia.

Certain indole derivatives, such as *oxypertine* and *molindone* appear to possess antipsychotic properties. Other dibenzyl structures including *clozapine* and *metiapine* have similar effects with less tendency to produce parkinsonian symptoms.

Drug treatment

Acute schizophrenia

An acute schizophrenic episode frequently presents with obvious delusory ideas, accompanied by auditory hallucinations. In addition there may be frank thought disorder with ideas of reference, ideas of influence and passivity feelings. Such a situation, whether arising for the first time, or resulting from a relapse in a patient who has had a similar illness in the past, calls for energetic medication with one of the neuroleptic drugs. This can be done either on an in-patient or an out-patient basis, although generally speaking the majority of patients suffering from acute schizophrenia will require in-patient treatment for a short time, particularly if they are disturbed in their behaviour.

1 *Initial control* Once the diagnosis of acute schizophrenia has been made, the next step is to decide on the choice of medication and the route of administration. If, as is usually the case, there is a certain amount of motor excitement, arising perhaps out of the patient's delusional fears, administration of a neuroleptic with sedative effects would be advisable. A phenothiazine with an aliphatic side-chain such as chlorpromazine is particularly suitable. It is difficult to be dogmatic about dosage but the following guidelines are suggested:

(i) In the case of a healthy male patient under the age of sixty, up to 300 mg of the drug may be given as a starting dose. This can be repeated as necessary up to four times in twenty-four hours for the first few days. In most cases it is usually possible to reduce the dosage to between 100 and 200 mg twice or four times daily within a short time. The physician will need to be guided on the one hand by the amount by which disturbed behaviour has been reduced and on the other hand by the degree of somnolence produced by the medication. It may be that the first dose produces so much drowsiness that the dosage can be sharply reduced almost immediately. Sometimes, however, even 300 mg of chlorpromazine proves inadequate to reduce the acute disturbance sufficiently and an even higher dosage may be required. In many cases with frank behaviour disturbance, the oral route is not possible and the drug has to be given intramuscularly. The dosage of chlorpromazine would be the same, but the addition of an equal amount of amylobarbitone sodium in the same syringe often produces a more satisfactory effect. Intramuscular administration is rarely required after the first 24–48 hours, as by then the patient has usually become sufficiently cooperative to take his drugs by mouth.

(ii) A healthy woman under the age of sixty should be given up to 200 mg chlorpromazine as a starting dose, otherwise the initial drug treatment is as outlined for a healthy male.

(iii) A patient who is known to be in frail physical health, or anyone over the age of sixty, should not be given more than 100 mg chlorpromazine in the first instance. Particular care should be taken in patients with cardiovascular abnormalities lest drug-induced hypotension should embarrass their circulation yet further. Similarly those with a known history of liver disease should be treated cautiously as they are often particularly sensitive to the central effects of phenothiazine compounds.

2 *Amelioration of schizophrenic symptoms* Once control of disturbed behaviour has been achieved the next step is to decide upon the most suitable treatment for the particular symptom complex present in the individual case. The symptoms most responsive to neuroleptic medication are paranoid delusions and auditory hallucinations; thought disorder, apathy and abnormalities of emotional response are less likely to improve so gratifyingly.

There is a bewildering choice of drugs available, all of which have been claimed to be useful in the management of schizophrenia. These include some ten phenothiazine compounds, four thioxanthene derivatives, at least three butyrophenones and three members of the closely related diphenylbutylpiperidines, plus a number of others (see Table 4)

Several well-conducted large-scale clinical trials have failed to reveal any significant differences in overall efficacy between one neuroleptic phenothiazine and another. Furthermore, although it had been suggested that those phenothiazine drugs with piperazine side-chains (e.g. trifluoperazine and fluphenazine) were more effective than the aliphatic phenothiazines (e.g. chlorpromazine) in stimulating apathetic schizophrenic patients into activity, the evidence obtained from the clinical trials fails to support this suggestion. The choice of drug depends more upon the side-effects produced, which vary from drug to drug, and upon the frequency of dosage required.

Chlorpromazine remains the standard medication in schizophrenia against which other treatments must be measured. It has been repeatedly shown to be more effective in schizophrenia than an inert placebo or an anxiolytic sedative such as phenobarbitone. It is also better than the antihistamine compound promethazine from which it was originally derived. With chlorpromazine over 60 per cent of patients with acute schizophrenic symptoms can be expected to improve significantly within a matter of weeks. The dosage of chlorpromazine required to achieve this varies considerably from case to case but is rarely less than 100 mg three times a day and may be as high as 300 mg four times daily. Once a steady state has been achieved it may be possible to reduce the dose by half without a recrudescence of symptoms. The drawbacks of chlorpromazine are its sedative effects and tendency to produce extrapyramidal symptoms (see below), together with the possibility of cholestatic jaundice, although the incidence of this seems to be falling. If over-sedation proves a problem in management with chlorpromazine then one of the piperazine compounds such as trifluoperazine (Stelazine) 5–10 mg or fluphenazine (Moditen, Prolixin) 2·5–5 mg three times daily may be tried. While they are certainly less sedating, they produce rather more extrapyramidal symptoms (see below). In contrast thioridazine (Melleril), 100–200 mg three times daily is the least likely of all the phenothiazines to cause such unwanted effects, but it, too, has its drawbacks. It is as sedative as chlorpromazine and is rather more likely to produce hypotension. In addition it interferes with ejaculation in men and may consequently prove unacceptable to many male patients if given over a period longer than a month or two, in addition there is the risk of producing retinal pigmentation.

Neither the thioxanthene derivatives nor the butyrophenones appear to have any advantage over the phenothiazines in the management of schizophrenia. The newer compounds in the diphenylbutylpiperidine group may prove to be more useful. Pimozide (Orap) requires only once daily administration. This is not only an advantage to the nurses in a busy psychiatric ward, but it also means that the prescribed dosage is more likely to be taken by the patient at home if he has to remember to take his pills only once during the day instead of three times. In this connection, however, it has recently been suggested that phenothiazine medication need only be given twice daily at most, once initial control has been obtained.

88

3 *Longer term medication* How long should one go on treating an acute episode of schizophrenia? There is no really clear-cut answer possible, for that depends on the presenting illness. If the episode is the first manifestation of schizophrenia in a particular patient of a previously good personality, and if there was no emotional abnormality during the illness, which itself was of acute onset and short duration, then the chances are that longer-term medication will not prove necessary. In a recent study it was found that among a group of such patients given no further medication after discharge from hospital the relapse rate was just over 25 per cent. When these criteria were not met, the relapse rate without further drug treatment among those who had responded reasonably well to treatment in the acute phase was over 80 per cent. In contrast, long-term treatment in this second group reduced the relapse rate to 33 per cent. Thus some patients will recover completely from acute schizophrenia and require no further drug treatment for the time being, whereas other patients never fully recover in the sense that they can remain symptom-free without medication. This latter group is often referred to as suffering from chronic schizophrenia, and management of this condition raises problems of its own.

Chronic schizophrenia

If after a first attack of schizophrenia the patient relapses shortly after his medication is stopped then it is likely that he is suffering from the chronic form of the condition and will require continuous medication for years, if not for life. While this need for long-term treatment may well be recognised by the medical advisers concerned with treatment, it is frequently not accepted by the patient. Consequent failure to take the medication leads to recrudescence of symptoms with readmission; in fact the most common cause for readmission to hospital is a relapse following failure to take the drugs prescribed.

As in the case of acute schizophrenia, no one neuroleptic drug stands out from the rest in terms of efficacy, provided the drug is taken. Several investigations have revealed how inconstant and unreliable many patients are in their medication. They stop it either because they feel well and can see no point in continuing, or because the side-effects are sufficiently unpleasant to deter them from persevering. Although such behaviour is by no means confined to schizophrenics (see chapter 3), it creates particularly severe management problems in them. What is required is some way of ensuring that schizophrenic patients take their medication for as long as is considered necessary. The introduction of the long-acting fluphenazine compounds fluphenazine enanthate (Moditen enanthate) and fluphenazine decanoate (Modecate) given by intramuscular injection every one to four weeks has gone a long way to meeting this requirement.

If, however, a patient is known to be reliable in taking oral medication, then there is no need to change his treatment regime to intramuscular injections. Only when it is considered unlikely that a particular patient is going to take his tablets conscientiously outside hospital is it advisable to stabilise him on a programme of fluphenazine injections before he is discharged. A test dose of 12·5 mg (0·5 ml) is usually given. If after a week no untoward reaction has occurred then a dose of 25 mg (1·0 ml) can be given. The administration requires some care: the drug must be given by deep intramuscular injection, preferably into the gluteal region. The most common untoward reaction is the development of extra-pyramidal symptoms (see below) which usually manifest themselves two to eight days after the injection. In addition, certain patients can become severely depressed during treatment with intramuscular long-acting fluphenazine; when this occurs, treatment with tricyclic antidepressant drugs as for depressive illness (see chapter 9) may help.

Flupenthixol decanoate (Depixol) 20–40 mg every one to three weeks is said not to cause depression; on the contrary, a definite antidepressant activity has been remarked upon by some observers.

Patients are usually asked to attend special clinics to receive their regular injections. This not only allows an efficient routine to be adopted by the patients and the nursing staff administering the fluphenazine injections, but it makes it easy to spot when a patient fails to attend. In that case he can either be asked to come up for his injection at another time, or, failing that, he can be visited in his home by a nurse who can given him the long-acting fluphenazine injection there and then. The adoption of such a treatment programme for patients with chronic schizophrenia discharged into the community has been shown to reduce the relapse rate dramatically. There are other injectable long-acting neuroleptics, such as fluspirilene, but they do not appear to possess any added advantages.

More recently a long-acting oral compound, penfluridol, has been developed. It is a member of the diphenylbutylpiperidine group of drugs. Preliminary reports suggest that oral administration once a week of penfluridol in a dose of 10–40 mg can maintain patients symptom-free. While penfluridol does away with the discomfort of injections it is not yet certain whether weekly oral medication will prove as reliable as regular injections.

The maintenance therapy of those chronic schizophrenic patients whose symptoms do not remit sufficiently for them to live outside hospital is not so difficult to control and supervise. Here the problem may be one of unnecessarily prolonged medication rather than its absence. These patients remain incapable of leading an independent life in spite of adequate neuroleptic treatment. In many cases stopping their drug does not lead to any deterioration in their condition; on the contrary there may be marked improvement associated with lessening of extrapyramidal symptoms. Even in those patients in whom continued medication is shown to be of benefit, a reduction in dosage may be achieved. Therefore, it is advisable to review from time to time the medication of all long-term in-patients receiving continuous neuroleptic therapy.

Unwanted effects of neuroleptic drugs

Extrapyramidal symptoms

These can be considered under four headings:

The first three are relatively acute, they are also clearly dose–dependent and disappear when medication ceases. The fourth group appears often to be irreversible, sometimes even getting worse after neuroleptic treatment has ceased.

Such reactions occur in up to 40 per cent of patients treated with phenothiazines, being more common with those compounds having a piperazine side-chain. They are equally frequent with butyrophenone medication.

1 *Pseudo-parkinsonism* The clinical picture mimics idiopathic parkinsonism very closely, with a general stiffening of the limbs, lack of facial expression, characteristic coarse tremor of the hands and head at rest, plus sialorrhoea and seborrhoea. This may even go on to a complete seizing up with a virtual absence of movement. Chlorpromazine is particularly prone to produce this syndrome.

2 *Akathisia* This condition of restlessness causes great distress to the patient, who feels he cannot keep still. This leads him to fidget continuously, shuffling up and down, or rocking his body backwards and forwards. This syndrome occurs most often with piperazine phenothiazines.

3 *Acute dyskinesias* These are more acute reactions, of which the oculogyric crisis is probably the best known. It begins with a fixed stare which then gives way to a turning upwards of the eyes followed by hyperextension of the neck and opening of the mouth. The attack may last several hours before subsiding spontaneously. The dyskinesic reactions can also involve the trunk or limb, producing grotesque postures or writhing movements, which are extremely distressing.

4 *Chronic tardive dyskinesia* This condition is characterised by virtually continuous movements of the head and tongue and certain postural changes. They may persist for years after all neuroleptic medication has been stopped. While they were originally thought to be particularly prevalent in patients with brain damage who had received phenothiazine medication in high dosage for years, this has now been shown not to be necessarily true. In fact some doubt has even been cast on the relationship to phenothiazines, as in one series at least 25 per cent of the patients with this condition had never received any neuroleptic drug.

The management of unwanted drug effects

Extrapyramidal reactions

The first step in the management of drug-induced pseudo-parkinsonism and akathisia is to stop the drug temporarily or sharply reduce the dose. Many patients will not deteriorate if their medication stops for a few days, particularly if they have been receiving it for several weeks. This measure, together with the administration of an anti-parkinsonian drug is usually sufficient. Of those available benzhexol (Artane) 2–4 mg, orphenadrine (Disipal) 50–100 mg, and methixene (Tremonil) 5–10 mg three times daily would appear to be equally effective; however, a recent trial has cast some doubt on their ability to influence the course of drug-induced parkinsonism. Contrary to the situation in idiopathic parkinsonism, laevo-dopa makes schizophrenic patients with phenothiazine-induced parkinsonism worse. However, a newer type of anti-parkinsonian agent, amantadine (which releases dopamine from neuronal stores), when given in a dose of 100–200 mg per day, may prove to be useful; but thus far clinical trials have not established its efficacy in drug-induced parkinsonism.

Acute dyskinesia responds best to parenteral biperiden (Akineton) given either by slow intravenous injection or intramuscularly in a dose of 2–5 mg.

We do not recommend the routine administration of anti-parkinsonian agents to all patients receiving neuroleptics. Not only may they be unnecessary, but also they produce other unwanted effects of their own, particularly anticholergenic symptoms which exacerbate the autonomic actions produced by the phenothiazines themselves.

Persistent chronic dyskinesia is much more resistant to treatment, although there are recent reports that tetrabenazine 25 mg three to four times daily may help. A phenothiazine compound, thiopropazate hydrochloride (Dartalan) has also been found useful in this condition.

Autonomic effects

1 *Antiadrenergic* Most phenothiazines have a marked anti-adrenergic activity. This is particularly true for those with a piperidine side-chain such as thioridazine. These can produce severe postural hypotension leading to circulatory collapse. Raising the foot of the bed is usually sufficient to restore cerebral circulation. In extreme cases noradrenaline (*not adrenaline*) should be given by intravenous infusion.

Other cardiovascular complications of phenothiazine medication include ECG changes and frank dysrhythmias which may go on to ventricular fibrillation. These are considered to be related to a quinidine-like action of the phenothiazines, particularly thioridazine.

Of less clinical importance, but causing extreme annoyance to patients when it does occur, is failure of ejaculation. This is also more commonly a consequence of thioridazine medication than of other phenothiazines. However, this effect may be put to good use in the treatment of patients presenting with premature ejaculation (see chapter 7).

2 *Anticholinergic* As a result of the anticholinergic action of the phenothiazines, dryness of the mouth, constipation, difficulty in micturition, and blurred vision can occur.

Metabolic effects

1 *Body weight* There is often considerable weight gain noted by patients on phenothiazines, particularly chlorpromazine. The pathogenesis of this is not known, but many patients report a marked increase in hunger, and this, together with the reduction in activity caused by the sedative effect of the drug, may well account for the gain in weight. This particular combination of effects is of value in the management of anorexia nervosa (see chapter 12). When it becomes troublesome a low-calorie diet should be instituted, and in some cases a non-stimulant appetite suppressant, such as fenfluramine (Ponderax) (see chapter 12) may be helpful.

2 *Endocrine* Phenothiazine drugs have been implicated as a cause of menstrual irregularity, and of lactation in non-pregnant women. Reduced libido or impotence can occur in the male.

3 *Pigmentation* Possibly as a result of the catalytic effect of ultra-violet light acting upon the melanin in the skin in the presence of phenothiazines, melanin may be deposited in the exposed skin. This leads to the purplish pigmentation in these areas which may be seen in patients receiving high doses of chlorpromazine for long periods. Melanin deposits may also be found in the cornea and in the lens of the eye. D-penicillamine in a dose of 1 g daily is said to be effective in reducing this pigmentation. In addition, thioridazine in high dosage can produce pigmentary retinopathy.

Convulsant activity

The epileptic seizure threshold is reduced by administration of phenothiazine drugs, and fits may occur even in patients without a previous epileptic history, while known epileptics show an increase in fit frequency.

Hypersensitivity reactions

1 *Cholestatic jaundice* Some patients receiving chlorpromazine develop jaundice of the cholestatic type within a few weeks of

starting medication. The incidence of the complication, at one time reported to be about 1 per cent of all patients given chlorpromazine, appears to have fallen considerably in recent years. When chlorpromazine-induced jaundice does occur the drug must be stopped immediately. The jaundice then nearly always subsides spontaneously within a few weeks. If necessary, another neuroleptic drug may be given when liver function has returned to normal.

2 *Leukopenia* A fall in the total white cell count which may progress to fatal agranulocytosis occurs in a tiny minority of patients on phenothiazines (perhaps one to four in every million patients). Unfortunately, when it does happen the onset is rapid; routine monitoring of the total white cell count is therefore unlikely to pick it up in time. Any patient on phenothiazines (particularly chlorpromazine) complaining of a sore throat or fever, should have an immediate haematological investigation. If a fall in the leucocyte count is found, the drug must be stopped straight away and a full course of antibiotic treatment begun. Even with energetic treatment the mortality rate may be as high as 50 per cent. If the patient survives, extreme caution should be taken before prescribing any neuroleptic drug again.

3 *Skin reactions* Urticarial sensitivity rashes are not uncommon after neuroleptic medication. In addition, light-sensitive dermatoses may lead to an erythematous response of the exposed skin, or a more serious eczematous rash. Protecting the skin from sunlight is the only sure way of avoiding complication. Barrier creams are of limited value.

Social implications of drug treatment in schizophrenia

At about the same time as the phenothiazines were being introduced into psychiatry the social climate inside large mental hospitals was changing rapidly. The old order of impersonal custodial care gave way to the concept of more direct involvement of the patient in his own environment, leading to the development of the 'therapeutic community'. Patients were encouraged to work, at first in the hospital in well-organised industrial rehabilitation units and later in the community, either in open employment, or failing that, in sheltered workshops where the work demands could be geared to the patients' abilities. These welcome changes in attitude towards schizophrenic patients have been considerably assisted by the development of neuroleptic drugs. While many of these changes would have taken place in any case, the symptomatic relief brought about by the neuroleptic drugs has allowed the resocialisation of chronic schizophrenic patients within the community to proceed at a faster pace, and to include a greater number than would have otherwise been possible. The social and pharmacological approaches in the management of schizophrenia should be considered as complementary rather than alternatives.

Table 4   *Neuroleptic drugs*

Approved name	Proprietary name	Recommended dose (daily unless stated otherwise)	Remarks
phenothiazines			
aliphatic side chain			
chlorpromazine	Largactil, Thorazine	Acutely disturbed patient: 300–900 mg Maintenance therapy: 100–500 mg	The standard phenothiazine. As effective as all other neuroleptics in the treatment of schizophrenia. But more marked tendency to produce drowsiness and risk of cholestatic jaundice and blood dyscrasias rather higher
promazine	Sparine	150–300 mg	Least effective of the phenothiazines, and more sedating. Useful for reducing disturbed behaviour in the elderly
trifluopromazine	Vesprin	20–100 mg	Equal to chlorpromazine in efficacy—no advantage over other phenothiazines
acepromazine	Notensil	50–300 mg	
propiomazine	Largon	10–40 mg	
methoxypromazine	Tentone		

Table 4—*Contd.*

Approved name	Proprietary name	Recommended dose (daily unless stated otherwise)	Remarks
piperidine side chain			
thioridazine	Melleril	150–600 mg	As effective as chlorpromazine with less tendency to produce extrapyramidal symptoms. More prone however to antiadrenergic effects such as hypotension and failure of ejaculation. Thioridazine can cause retinal pigmentation in prolonged dosage
mesoridazine	Serentil	100–300 mg	
piperacetazine	Quide	25–100 mg	
piperazine side chain			More extrapyramidal effects than other phenothiazines
prochlorperazine	Stemetil	25–150 mg	The piperazine analogue of chlorpromazine to which it is clinically equivalent but produces decreased rather than increased appetite
trifluoperazine	Stelazine	10–30 mg	No advantages over other phenothiazines
thiethylperazine	Torecan	10–30 mg	Potent antiemetic
thioproperazine	Majeptil	10–40 mg	High incidence of extrapyramidal symptoms
butaperazine	Repoise	30–100 mg	No obvious advantages over other phenothiazines
perphenazine	Fentazin Trilafon	12–24 mg	
fluphenazine	Moditen Prolixin	2·5–15 mg	

Table 4—*Contd.*

Approved name	*Proprietary name*	*Recommended dose (daily unless stated otherwise)*	*Remarks*
fluphenazine enanthate	Moditen enanthate	12·5–25 mg every 1–3 weeks	Long-acting form given by deep intramuscular injection. Very useful in out-patient maintenance therapy of chronic schizophrenia
fluphenazine decanoate	Modecate	12·5–25 mg every 2–4 weeks	
thiopropazate	Dartalan Dartal	15–30 mg	Equal in efficacy to chlorpromazine. May relieve symptoms of persistent dyskinesia
pericyazine	Neulactil	7·5–90 mg	Said to be useful in the management of character disorders
metho-trimeprazine	Veractil	15–100 mg	No obvious advantage over the other phenothiazines
acetophenazine	Tindal	40–80 mg	
carphenazine	Proketazine	40–400 mg	

thioxanthenes

chlorprothixene	Taractan	50–300 mg	Thioxanthene analogue of chlorpromazine. Possibly slightly inferior to chlorpromazine in acute schizophrenia
clopenthixol	Sordinol	100–400 mg	Thioxanthene analogue of perphenizine to which it may be equal in efficacy, although also said to be inferior to chlorpromazine
thiothixene	Navane	10–30 mg	Thioxanthene analogue of thioproperazine. As effective as phenothiazines but prone to cause extrapyramidal effects

Table 4—*Contd.*

Approved name	Proprietary name	Recommended dose (daily unless stated otherwise)	Remarks
flupenthixol	Fluanxol	3–12 mg	Thioxanthene analogue of fluphenazine to which it is equal in efficacy
flupenthixol decanoate	Depixol	20–40 mg every 1–3 weeks	Long-acting form of flupenthixol useful for maintenance therapy of chronic schizophrenia. Possibly less likely to cause depression than fluphenazine decanoate
indole derivatives			
oxypertine	Integrin	20–60 mg	Equal to phenothiazines in efficacy in schizophrenia. Effective in lower dose in treatment of anxiety
molindone	——	10–20 mg	Possibly slower-acting than phenothiazines in acute schizophrenia
dibenzodiazepines clozapine	Leponex	150–300 mg	Effective in schizophrenia, causes few extrapyramidal effects, but can produce marked hypotension
dibenzothiazepine metiapin	——	100–300 mg	
benzoquinolizine			
tetrabenazine	Nitoman	75–150 mg	Less effective than chlorpromazine in schizophrenia. May be useful in tardive dyskinesia

99

Table 4—*Contd.*

Approved name	Proprietary name	Recommended dose (daily unless stated otherwise)	Remarks
butyrophenones			
haloperidol	Serenace Haldol	1–12 mg	As effective as pheno-thiazines in schizo-phrenia, but very prone to cause extrapyramidal symptoms. Said to be particularly effective in mania. In low dosage may help in anxiety
trifluperidol (triperidol)	Triperidol	1–3 mg	Possibly among the most effective neuroleptics, having been shown to be superior to chlorpro-mazine, but not to trifluoperazine
benperidol (benzperidol)	Frenactil	2–6 mg	Less effective than chlorpromazine in schizophrenia. Appears to reduce sexual drive, and thus may be of some use in the treatment of sexual offenders
diphenylbutyl-piperidines			
pimozide	Orap	2–8 mg	As effective as pheno-thiazines in schizo-phrenia. Main advantage is that it only needs to be given once daily. Few side-effects, but may lead to an increase in aggression
fluspirilene	Imap	2–6 mg weekly	Long-acting compound. Administered once weekly by intramuscular injection. Used in maintenance therapy of chronic schizophrenia

Table 4—*Contd.*

Approved name	Proprietary name	Recommended dose (daily unless stated otherwise)	Remarks
penfluridol	Semap	20–50 mg weekly	Long-acting oral compound—apparently one weekly dose affords adequate maintenance therapy in chronic schizophrenia but tends to produce extra-pyramidal symptoms

Suggestions for further reading

BOBON, D. P., JANSSEN, P. A. J., and BOBON, J., *The Neuroleptics*, Karger, Basel, 1970.

COPPEN, A., and WALK, A., 'Recent developments in schizophrenia', *British Journal of Psychiatry*, Special Publication, No. 1, 1967.

FISH, F. J., *Schizophrenia*, Wright, Bristol, 1962.

HIMWICH, H., *Biochemistry, Schizophrenia and Affective Illnesses*, Williams & Wilkins, Baltimore, 1970.

LEFF, J., 'Maintenance therapy and schizophrenia', *British Journal of Hospital Medicine*, Vol. 8, pp. 377–80, 1972.

6 Affective disorders

Introduction

The affective disorders are those conditions in which there is alteration of mood to such a degree as to cause serious distress or disruption of normal life. The mood may be abnormally elevated as in mania, or lowered as in depression. Depression may either be a symptom of reaction to adverse circumstances, or an illness in its own right. The tendency to confuse the symptom with the illness has in the past led to certain conceptual difficulties. We all get depressed (symptom) from time to time when things go wrong; this is a perfectly natural reaction. Some people react rather more frequently and sharply than others, but the quality of their *depressive reaction* does not differ from our own. A few people, however, (1–2 per cent of the population) develop a much more serious condition—a true *depressive illness* which, as often as not, comes completely out of the blue with no obvious precipitating cause. A number of labels have been given to this illness: 'melancholia', 'psychotic depression', 'the depressive phase of a manic-depressive psychosis', 'endogenous depression', and, when it comes on later in life, 'involutional melancholia'. Essentially, however, they are all similar in their manifestation and the basic treatment approach is the same for each. Only when states of depression alternate with episodes of mania should the term manic-depressive psychosis be used. Some authors refer to the depressive phase of this particular variant as 'bipolar' depression, reserving 'unipolar' depression for those cases in which mania has not previously appeared.

Psychopathology

Depressive illness

This can be described as a persistent alteration of mood, exceeding customary sadness, which characteristically comes on 'out of the blue' with no obvious environmental precipitant. It is usually accompanied by one or more of the following symptoms: self-deprecation and a morbid sense (or delusional ideas) of guilt; sleep disturbance (typically early morning awakening); retardation of thought or action; agitated behaviour; suicidal ideas or attempts at suicide; an inability to concentrate and lack of interest in the surroundings; profound anorexia with consequent weight loss. It does not change with alteration in environmental circumstance and requires treatment with drugs or electroconvulsive therapy (ECT).

Depressive reaction

This, on the other hand, can clearly be seen to arise as the direct result of some unfortunate circumstance in the patient's life. Typically the patient blames others for his misfortune rather than himself. (In contrast, the patient with depressive illness is usually riddled with self-blame.) In a depressive reaction there are no delusional ideas, severe retardation is uncommon and successful suicide occurs far less frequently. The sleep disturbance is characteristically a difficulty in getting off to sleep rather than early morning waking. Although anorexia may occur in some patients, others turn to food for comfort and thus gain, rather than lose, weight. Finally, depressive reactions readily respond to environmental changes, and if the precipitating circumstances can be alleviated further treatment often proves unnecessary.

Mania

Mania occurs less frequently than depression. It is characterised by over-activity both day and night, loss of social inhibitions and lack of judgment leading to self-assertiveness, over-generosity and recklessness. In addition, the manic patient has a sense of well-being and talks non-stop in a continuous stream of jokes, puns and personal remarks, which very soon become extremely wearisome to the listener. While some cases abort spontaneously, most require medical intervention.

Biochemical basis of affective disorders

Both depressive illness and mania are associated with biochemical changes in the brain and other parts of the body which are of importance in pathogenesis and in the further development of the disorder. These changes involve particularly the brain amines, the electrolytes sodium and potassium, and certain hormones, particularly thyroid and adrenocorticosteroid hormones.

Monoamines

Increasing interest in the role of monoamines, such as noradrenaline, dopamine and 5HT, in depressive illness followed the introduction of antidepressant drugs. These drugs were found to have an effect on brain monoamine metabolism, to which their therapeutic effect was attributed. The monoamine oxidase inhibitors (MAOI) increase the levels of brain monoamines by inhibiting their metabolism by MAO. Although this inhibition is seen within a few hours of administration in animals, in man, where smaller doses are given, it may take two to three weeks before the levels of brain 5HT and noradrenaline begin to rise. It may be of significance that this period is similar to that taken for the maximum antidepressant effect to appear clinically.

The dibenzazepine drugs (tricyclic antidepressants) are another group of antidepressant compounds which have been shown to potentiate the peripheral and central actions of noradrenaline and 5HT. Their mechanism of action is probably to inhibit uptake of noradrenaline and 5HT into neuronal tissue so increasing their activity at central receptor sites. Even though the total brain level of monoamines is not increased, the rate of turnover probably is. In contrast to these drugs, which possess antidepressant properties, by virtue of increased brain monoamine activity, are reserpine and tetrabenazine which may produce serious depression by depleting the brain of catecholamines and 5HT. Such observations have provided a basis for the monoamine theory of affective disorders which may be stated as follows:

(i) Depression is due to an absolute or relative *decrease* in monoamines at receptor sites in the brain, while mania is due to an absolute or relative *excess* of monoamines at these receptors.
(ii) Successful treatment of these conditions depends on restoring to normal monoamine activity at the central receptor sites.

The relative importance of noradrenaline, dopamine and 5HT in the monoamine theory has not yet been established. The MAOIs and dibenzazepines affect the metabolism or uptake of all three monoamines, and although some drugs in both groups appear to influence one amine more than another in experimental animals, it is not possible to extrapolate their actions to man. Conversely, reserpine depletes both catecholamines and 5HT, and the sedation and depression which it produces may be associated with reduction of the intracerebral concentration of one or all of these amines. Changes in urinary excretion and in CSF concentration of both catecholamine and 5HT metabolites in clinical states of mania and depression have been described by independent groups of investigators. In some animal species administration of dopa, the precursor of dopamine and noradrenaline, reverses reserpine-induced sedation, suggesting that catecholamines play a major role. Other studies, however, have shown that catecholamines may be reduced to as much as 20 per cent of the normal level without producing sedation, provided that brain 5HT is maintained within the normal range. Further evidence indicating the importance of 5HT in man is the potentiation of the antidepressant effect of an MAOI by tryptophan, a precursor of 5HT. A variant of this hypothesis has been put forward by Kety who suggests that a fall in cerebral 5HT levels 'permits' affective change to occur, but in itself is not sufficient; in addition a change in catecholamine level is needed to produce the clinical syndrome; a fall in catecholamines leads to depression and a rise produces mania.

As an alternative to the monoamine theory, Dewhurst and Marley have proposed a hypothesis to account for the role of noradrenaline and 5HT in terms of central receptors. They classified monoamines into central excitant and central depressant groups, and pointed out that the excitant amines (Type A) had the general formula $R.CH_2.CH_2.NH_2$, where R is a fat-soluble planar hydrocarbon such as an indolyl or phenyl group. These amines, of which tryptamine is the most potent, produce behavioural and physiological excitation in immature chicks (chosen because the blood-brain barrier is not established in them) probably by activation of specific central receptors. Depressant amines (Type C) are of general structure $R'CH(OH)CH_2.NH.CH_3$ where R' is water soluble (e.g. catechol). Such amines, of which adrenaline is the most potent, produce drowsiness or sleep in the immature chick, and are thought to act through other receptors. It would appear that the type of receptor action of a particular compound depends primarily on its lipid solubility. If this hypothesis is correct, then a specific antagonist of the Type A (excitant) amines should reduce excitation and be effective in mania. Methysergide is a potent antitryptamine drug, and, in fact, in some studies, although not all, has been claimed to control manic disorders rapidly and effectively. While this lends weight to the Dewhurst and Marley hypothesis, serious objections to it remain. For example, adrenaline does not produce sedation in man, but excitation, and it is by no means certain that this is only of peripheral rather than central origin. It is, in fact, probably an over-simplification to suggest that noradrenaline and 5HT have such opposing actions in man, particularly on the basis of experimental work done in the chick. It is more likely that they have both excitant and inhibitory effects on different groups of neurones and that satisfactory treatment of affective disorders depends on restoring a normal balance of these actions. Furthermore, other transmitters such as dopamine may play an equally important part which has yet to be defined. It is also possible that different types of manic or depressive disorder are associated with changes in one monoamine rather than another. For instance, the CSF levels of both 5-hydroxyindoleacetic acid, (5HIAA) (the breakdown product of 5HT), and homovanilic acid (HVA) (derived from dopamine) were found to be lower than normal in patients with unipolar depression, but not in those with bipolar depression. Furthermore, the levels did not rise with clinical recovery. On the basis of this and similar findings, Ashcroft has suggested that depression may result from either a reduction in monoamine output (as in unipolar depression) or by a reduction in post-synaptic receptor sensitivity (as in bipolar depression). Mania, on the other hand, might be a consequence of increased receptor sensitivity. It is the balance between transmitter availability and receptor sensitivity which is thought to be critical. The recent finding that thyrotropic hormones, which may affect receptor sensitivity directly, potentiate the action of tricyclic antidepressant drugs, is consistent with this hypothesis.

It could be, however, that many of the observed changes in monoamine levels may be secondary rather than primary; simulation of a manic state can lead to increase in the CSF levels of both 5HIAA and HVA.

Finally, the possible involvement of cholinergic neurones should not be overlooked. Blockade of central choline sterase with physostigmine can produce lethargy and dysphoria in normal subjects; similar treatment in patients with mania ameliorates their symptoms.

Electrolytes

In 1932 Gjessing showed that changes in water and electrolyte balance accompanied cyclic affective disorders in some patients. Since that time numerous studies have been carried out with conflicting results, because, although marked changes were demonstrated, no consistent pattern was associated with particular mental states in different patients.

The distribution of electrolytes in the cells and extracellular fluid has a profound influence on neuronal activity with the resting potential dependent on the ratio of the concentration of potassium inside and outside the cell, and the action potential dependent on the ratio of the concentrations of intracellular to extracellular sodium. Calcium and magnesium ions also have marked effects on nerve cell membranes and on release of neurotransmitters. It would not be surprising, therefore, if changes in concentration and distribution of electrolytes throughout the body, and particularly in the brain, were associated with changes in neuronal function and were reflected in disorders of behaviour and mood.

Evidence to support the belief that electrolytes do play a role in the pathogenesis of the affective disorders comes from the finding that lithium salts appear to have a prophylactic value in reducing the incidence and severity of recurrent mania and depression. It is not unlikely that these effects depend on its marked action on sodium transport across cell membranes, which change the distribution of sodium and chloride between the intra- and extracellular fluid spaces.

Endocrine function

While profound psychological changes may accompany all endocrine disorders, thyroid and adrenal cortical dysfunction in particular are associated with changes in mood. It is possible that thyroid hormone influences central nervous activity through changes in adenylcyclase, an enzyme identical to, or closely related to, the adrenergic receptor. Thyroid hormone stimulates adenylcyclase, which in turn leads to an increase in cyclic AMP. It is reasonable to suppose that changes in concentration of adenylcyclase and cyclic AMP in the brain may underlie some if not all of the psychological changes associated with a deficiency or excess of thyroid hormone.

A relationship between depression and adrenal cortical activity is suggested first by the clinical observation that states of profound depression may be produced by administration of high doses of corticotrophin or cortisol. Second, patients with severe endogenous depression may themselves frequently have raised plasma cortisol levels throughout the 24 hours, with a loss of normal diurnal variation. This is probably due, in turn, to an increased pituitary corticotrophin production which may depend on disordered hypothalamic control of anterior pituitary function.

Amine metabolism, electrolyte balance and thyroid and adrenal cortical function are all interrelated, and it is not yet possible to say whether changes in one or more of them are responsible for, or the result of, an affective disorder. If the monoamine hypothesis, or a variant of it, is correct then it might be envisaged that alterations in electrolyte distribution would modify neuronal excitability and transmitter release and uptake. Changes in neuronal activity in the hypothalamus might influence pituitary and adrenal cortical function to change the rate of cortisol production which in turn would produce further changes in electrolyte balance. Changes in thyroid function could modify monoamine activity, as has already been said, by altering brain levels of adenylcyclase and cyclic AMP. However, the way in which these biochemical events are linked to changes in mood and affect remains unknown.

Pharmacology

Central stimulant drugs

Before the development of the MAOI and tricyclic antidepressants, many cases of depression were treated with drugs which had a central stimulating effect. The use of these drugs in depression is now becoming much less; their short-term effects on mood do however throw some light on the possible biochemical basis of affective disorders.

1   *Xanthines* Xanthine derivatives such as caffeine, theophylline and theobromine are central stimulant compounds, which prevent the impairment of performance produced by muscular fatigue, deprivation of sleep or boredom. The capacity for physical exertion is augmented, but recently acquired motor skills requiring careful co-ordination may be impaired. Excessive administration produces insomnia, restlessness, anxiety, headache and tremor. Dependence

on these compounds can develop, and a characteristic withdrawal syndrome may be seen with fatigue, depression, headache and irritability.

Although they increase central nervous activity, xanthines do not restore normality of mood in patients with endogenous depression, and cannot be considered to be true antidepressant drugs. Their mechanism of action depends on inhibition of the enzyme phosphodiesterase which is responsible for the inactivation of cyclic AMP which is thought to be intimately involved with adrenergic receptor activity. Phosphodiesterase inhibition, by increasing cyclic AMP activity, produces effects similar to adrenergic stimulation. The central effects of xanthines are therefore consistent with the monoamine theory as far as it relates to changes in noradrenaline receptor activity.

2 *Sympathomimetic amines* The indirectly acting sympathomimetic amines, such as amphetamine and phenmetrazine, probably produce excitation by release of catecholamines from, and blockade of uptake into, cortical neurones. Their central stimulant effect is seen in an increase of alertness and in motor and psychological activity, together with a decrease in fatigue and varying degrees of insomnia. These actions have led to their widespread abuse, and they are now subject to legal restrictions in many countries. Chronic use in large doses may ultimately lead to dangerous psychotic behaviour with paranoid features. As with the xanthine derivatives, their central effects lead to anxiety, restlessness and agitation rather than to a normality of mood, and they cannot be considered therapeutically useful antidepressant drugs. This may be because, like the xanthines, they enhance central adrenergic activity without increasing activity of 5HT.

Antidepressant compounds

1 *Monoamine oxidase inhibitors* (*MAOI*) Inhibition of the intracellular enzyme monoamine oxidase (MAO) leads to an increase of the monoamines noradrenaline, dopamine and 5HT in the brain. Any antidepressant effect MAO inhibitors may have would fit in well with the monoamine hypothesis. Many other drugs inhibit MAO to a limited extent, including cocaine and amphetamine, but their pharmacological actions do not appear to depend on this effect. The compounds in which antidepressant

effects probably depend on MAO inhibition fall into two chemical groups: (i) those which are hydrazine derivatives, particularly toxic to the liver (isocarboxazid, nialamide and phenelzine) and (ii) those related to amphetamine, the most important being tranyl-cypromine which appears to have intrinsic sympathomimetic activity of its own. Some of this latter group of drugs, particularly tranylcypromine are also potent inhibitors of noradrenaline uptake. It is, therefore, uncertain to what extent an increased level of noradrenaline at the receptor site produced by tranylcypromine is due to inhibition of metabolic degradation of noradrenaline on the one hand and to inhibition of uptake on the other.

Monoamine oxidase is not a single entity but a group of more specific enzymes, each of which is concerned with an individual monoamine. Most of the monoamine oxidase inhibitors in general use inhibit the whole family of enzymes and thus lead to an increase in all the monoamines. However, certain MAOI, such as clorgy-line, have been claimed, on the basis of animal experiments, to inhibit preferentially the enzyme responsible for one monoamine rather than another; but clinical pharmacological studies in man have failed to demonstrate this selectivity of action.

MAO is important in the handling of many drugs and foodstuffs within the body. For this reason, drugs which inhibit the enzyme complex may have important interactions with it.

(a) *Sympathomimetic amines* After MAO inhibition, the in-directly acting amines may evoke enhanced effects both peri-pherally and centrally. Many easily available proprietary remedies for upper respiratory tract infections contain such amines, and thus patients taking MAO inhibitors must be cautious in their use.

(b) *Certain foodstuffs* Foods which contain pressor amines such as dopa and tyramine may produce hypertensive reactions in patients receiving MAO inhibitors. These include broad beans, which contain dopa, and certain cheeses containing large quantities of tyramine. Under normal circumstances most tyramine ingested by mouth is metabolised immediately by MAO in the intestinal mucosa and liver. Following MAO inhibition, the absorption of tyramine is increased markedly and it rapidly enters the circulation to cause prolonged release of noradrenaline and thus evoke pressor effects. Some wines, yeast products and animal livers also contain significant amounts of tyramine.

(c) *Central nervous depressant drugs* The central effects of pethidine and other narcotic compounds are prolonged in patients receiving MAOI, and excitation, rigidity, coma, changes in blood pressure, hyperpyrexia and shock may occur. This interaction can be prevented in animals by drugs such as p-chlorophenylalanine which prevent the intracerebral accumulation of 5HT but not by compounds which reduce noradrenaline synthesis. It appears, therefore, that an increase in brain 5HT is necessary for this interaction to occur.

(d) *Antihypertensive drugs* Some of the antihypertensive drugs, including guanethidine and bethanidine, may release noradrenaline from peripheral sympathetic nerve endings when administered in high concentration, for example, intravenously. In the absence of MAO activity, these compounds may release increased amounts of noradrenaline on to receptor sites and produce hyperexcitation and hypertension.

(e) *Dibenzazepine compounds* These antidepressant drugs, such as imipramine, as will be described later, inhibit uptake of noradrenaline and possibly 5HT into central nerve terminals, thus increasing their activity at receptor sites. It would be expected on theoretical grounds, therefore, that MAO inhibitors might potentiate their effects, and this has been demonstrated in animal experiments. There have also been reports of serious reactions in patients treated with a combination of these two groups of compounds.

2 *Dibenzazepines* (tricyclic antidepressant drugs) The dibenzazepine drugs have many pharmacological properties including anticholinergic, anti-5HT, antihistamine, hypothermic and antiemetic actions. Their antidepressant activity, however, is probably due to their ability to block the neuronal uptake of catecholamines and 5HT thus increasing the effective concentrations of these monoamines at central receptor sites, even though the brain amine content is not increased. It is probable that these compounds have both an acute action and a longer term, chronic action. After a single dose these drugs inhibit the uptake of noradrenaline and 5HT in the brain, and may also prevent deamination by MAO in the mitochondria. After tricyclic drugs have been administered to experimental animals for several days the uptake of monoamines is still reduced, and the levels of their metabolites are also reduced (as after acute administration). In contrast to the acute experiments, their rate of disappearance was *not* reduced, suggesting an increased turnover.

It may be that it is the delayed increase in rate of monoamine turnover which underlies the therapeutic activity of these drugs, which does not usually come on until ten days after administration. A further suggestion has been made that in order for these longer-term effects to take place enzyme synthesis is required, thus accounting for the delay.

Tricyclic antidepressant compounds also have a potent anticholinergic action; this too may be related to their clinical effect, particularly if there is a disturbance in the central cholinergic activity in depressive illness, as has recently been suggested. Imipramine is the parent compound of the group, and is metabolised within the body to its demethyl derivative desipramine. Several other dibenzazepines have been introduced and it is claimed on the basis of animal studies that some possess selectivity of action in blocking the uptake of one monoamine rather than another; tricyclic compounds of the secondary amine type (e.g. desipramine, protriptyline) are more potent than those of the tertiary amine type (e.g. imipramine, amitriptyline) in blocking NA uptake, whereas the tertiary amines are more potent in blocking 5HT uptake. If this is confirmed in man it may elucidate further the relative importance of noradrenaline and 5HT in the pathogenesis of endogenous depression.

The dibenzazepines also potentiate the peripheral pressor effect of noradrenaline and adrenaline as well as their central effects. This is particularly important in patients given injections of local anaesthetic preparations containing these catecholamines as vasoconstrictor agents. Another important interaction is with antihypertensive drugs such as guanethidine and bethanidine which block noradrenaline release after being taken up into the adrenergic neurone. The uptake of these drugs, like that of noradrenaline, is blocked by the dibenzazepines, and so their antihypertensive effect is reduced or abolished. The possible interaction of monoamine oxidase inhibitors with dibenzazepines has already been mentioned.

Recent reports have indicated that thyroid hormones and thyroid-releasing factors can markedly potentiate the action of tricyclic antidepressants, increasing both their efficacy and their speed of action, possibly by increasing receptor sensitivity to monoamines, the reuptake of which is blocked by the tricyclic antidepressant. In women, oestrogens have also been found to potentiate tricyclic antidepressant activity; this may be related to the reported increase in plasma monoamine oxidase levels in premenopausal depressed women, which would in turn lead to a reduction of catecholamine and 5HT. Therapy with oestrogens restores the plasma MAO level to normal.

Other drugs interfere with the metabolism of tricyclic antidepressants and thus influence their clinical effects. Phenothiazine compounds, such as chlorpromazine (see chapter 5) block their hydroxylation, thereby increasing the plasma level and potentiating their antidepressant activity (side-effects are increased as well). The central-stimulant drug, methylphenidate, has a similar action (although d-amphetamine does not).

Most tricylic compounds appear to have a direct action on the heart; they produce tachycardia (probably due to their anticholinergic activity) and may cause bundle branch block, or even complete heart block. They have been implicated in a number of unexpected cardiac deaths.

ECT Electroconvulsive therapy (ECT) still remains the most effective form of antidepressant treatment for severe cases. If the monoamine theory is true, then it would be expected that this form of treatment should also influence central monoamine activity. Its effect on cerebral amines in man are not known, but animal studies have shown a reduction in brain levels of noradrenaline in ECT-treated animals compared with untreated controls, suggesting that this procedure may increase neuronal discharge of noradrenaline in the brain. Furthermore, normetadrenaline levels were higher than in the controls, and as this metabolite is the result of COMT activity this would indicate an increased extraneuronal breakdown after release onto receptors.

Drugs in mania

1 *Phenothiazines* The pharmacology of these drugs is dealt with more fully elsewhere (see chapter 5). Their effectiveness in controlling mania may be explained in terms of the monoamine theory, by their ability to block adrenergic receptors. In the peripheral vascular system chlorpromazine reduces the hypertensive action of adrenaline and noradrenaline; it probably has similar effects in the central nervous system. In addition it possesses anti-5HT and antidopamine properties, which may also contribute to its therapeutic effects in mania.

2 *Butyrophenones* These drugs, which are more fully described elsewhere (see chapter 5) resemble the phenothiazines in their pharmacological actions. In particular, they block the central effects of catecholamines including dopamine and noradrenaline, and their effectiveness in mania is therefore consistent with the monoamine theory.

3 *Reserpine* The effectiveness of reserpine in controlling mania may be explained by the general monoamine depletion which it produces.

4 *Methysergide* Methysergide is a specific 5HT receptor blocking drug, and if its postulated antimanic action could be substantiated it would indicate that 5HT plays an important part in producing the manic state. It would also be consistent with the theory put forward by Dewhurst and Marley which suggested that tryptamine derivatives possess potent central stimulant properties which could be prevented by specific tryptamine-blocking drugs such as methysergide. Unfortunately for this hypothesis, controlled trials have thus far failed to support the use of methysergide in mania.

5 *Lithium* Lithium appears to be of value in the prophylactic treatment of mania, reducing or abolishing recurrence of manic episodes. In animals it displaces sodium from body fluids, and may substitute for sodium in nerve and skeletal muscle. Clinical studies in man have shown a triphasic pattern of water and electrolyte response. At first lithium causes a marked increase in urinary excretion of water and sodium, and less marked increases in potassium and calcium. This is followed by a compensatory retention of sodium, and finally there is a return to a stable normal state. Such electrolyte changes might be expected to modify central nervous activity and be responsible for its therapeutic effect. There is evidence, however, that lithium increases the intraneuronal deamination of noradrenaline with a decreased production of normetadrenaline. Furthermore, it appears that lithium diminishes the release of brain monoamines, in part, through interference with calcium participation in stimulus–release coupling. These actions would reduce the amount of free noradrenaline at central receptor sites and explain, in terms of the monoamine theory, any usefulness it may have in mania.

Treatment

Depression

When presented with a patient who is unhappy, perhaps weeping, obviously distressed, and who gives a history of inability to cope, a sense of hopelessness perhaps with suicidal ideas, profound anorexia and marked insomnia, it is necessary to determine first of all the likely underlying cause for these symptoms, and secondly to assess their severity. Treatment varies considerably according to the type of condition present (i.e. whether it is a true depressive illness or a depressive reaction to distressing circumstances), and to its severity. If the patient is so desperate that there is a real risk of a suicide attempt, or if he is so incapacitated by his symptoms as to be unable to care for himself adequately, hospitalisation is likely to be necessary, followed by treatment with electroconvulsive therapy (ECT). Where the patient is neither suicidal nor incapacitated, it will usually be possible to treat him with the appropriate medication as an out-patient. Although in many cases it is not possible to distinguish categorically between a depressive illness and a depressive reaction, an attempt to do so should be made, as the treatment is different for each. Depressive illness usually responds well to one of the tricyclic antidepressant drugs, whereas depressive reactions often respond more rapidly to an anxiolytic sedative rather than an antidepressant. Where the distinction between depressive illness and reaction cannot be made with any confidence, treatment should proceed as for depressive illness. In cases of so-called 'atypical' depression, particularly if there is a lengthy history, with failure to respond to tricyclic antidepressants, monoamine oxidase inhibitors may prove effective.

Depressive illness (endogenous depression)

1 *Tricyclic antidepressants* As we have already indicated, the treatment of first choice for depressive illness of mild to moderate severity is a tricyclic antidepressant. Imipramine (Tofranil), the first of these drugs to be introduced, was found by Kuhn to produce elation in the schizophrenic patients to whom it had been given. (As it structurally resembled chlorpromazine it was originally thought to be a neuroleptic compound, hence its administration to schizophrenic patients.) Following this, a considerable

number of related compounds have been synthesised and marketed for the treatment of depressive illness (see Table 5). In general some 60 to 70 per cent of depressed patients improve on tricyclic antidepressants (as compared to 30–40 per cent who improve on placebo and 70–80 per cent who improve on ECT). Patients who respond best are those suffering from a clear-cut depressive illness of moderate severity, with a history of less than six months' duration. As a rule the tricyclic antidepressants take some ten to fourteen days to become fully effective and the maximum response often does not occur for some three to four weeks after the start of treatment (an exception being protriptyline which appears to act more rapidly—see below). Among the factors which influence the metabolism and plasma levels of these drugs, and hence their efficacy, are genetic factors, other drugs being administered at the same time (particularly barbiturate and phenothiazine compounds), and pH (acidification of the urine leading to faster excretion).

In general all the members of this group of drugs have similar side-effects, the commonest being due to the pronounced anticholinergic properties they possess. These effects include dryness of the mouth, excessive sweating, postural hypotension which may lead to falling, difficulty in visual accommodation, constipation and urine retention. More dangerous are the cardiovascular effects. It is not uncommon to find a prolonged QT interval in the electrocardiogram in patients being treated with tricyclic antidepressants. This can proceed to a frank dysrhythmia or ventricular tachycardia, which in cases of overdose occasionally progresses to fatal ventricular fibrillation. In the elderly, congestive cardiac failure is not uncommon. In addition to these autonomic and cardiac effects, the tricyclics are epileptogenic and may precipitate epileptic seizures in those who are otherwise predisposed. In view of all these possible side-effects, tricyclic antidepressant drugs should be used most cautiously in patients with glaucoma, prostatism, chronic heart disease and epilepsy.

Chemically the majority of tricyclic antidepressants fall into two categories: (i) the iminodibenzyl sub-group of the dibenzazepines (e.g. imipramine) (ii) the dibenzocycloheptenes (e.g. amitriptyline). The choice of drug to use in any particular case depends on a number of factors. Efficacy is similar for all the marketed products (see Table 5 for effective dose regimes for individual drugs). Where they differ is in speed of action, sedative effects and side-effects.

The most rapidly acting tricyclic antidepressant is protriptyline (Concordin). As it acts within five days, as compared to the ten to fourteen days which imipramine takes to act, it has a pronounced advantage over the other tricyclic antidepressants when speed of action is important. (It had been hoped that the demethylated metabolite of imipramine, desipramine (Pertofran) would act more quickly than the parent compound. Unfortunately this proved not to be the case.)

Protriptyline produces marked autonomic effects which some patients are unable to tolerate. Such side-effects appear to be less with dothiepin (Prothiaden) and iprindole (Prondol) and they are consequently better tolerated, particularly by the elderly. However, iprindole medication has been followed by frank jaundice in a number of patients and signs of hepatatoxicity must therefore be closely watched for when it is prescribed.

Some patients exhibit overwhelming anxiety and restless agitation during the course of a depressive illness. In such cases it is obviously an advantage to have a compound which, in addition to its antidepressant activity, has a pronounced sedative effect. Amitriptyline (Tryptizol, Elavil), together with its oxepin and thiapin analogues, doxepin (Sinequan) and dothiepin (Prothiaden), do have this combination of actions and are thus particularly useful in the anxious, depressed patient. While there are also a variety of mixtures combining an antidepressant with an anxiolytic sedative (amitriptyline with chlordiazepoxide [Limbitrol]; amitriptyline with perphenazine [Triptafen]; imipramine with promazine), we would not recommend their use. If the addition of an anxiolytic sedative is thought necessary then one of the benzodiazepine group of drugs (see chapter 7) can be prescribed as required, allowing a greater flexibility of dosage.

The other tricyclic compounds listed in Table 5 would not appear to have any distinct advantages over those already discussed. It is better to become familiar with the dosage and effects of some two or three compounds and stick to them; for instance imipramine as the standard antidepressant, amitriptyline or one of its analogues (see above) for the patient with endogenous depression who is also anxious, dothiepin or iprindole when autonomic side-effects need to be reduced to a minimum, and protriptyline when a rapid onset of action is particularly important. The addition of liothyronine, 20 μg daily to treatment with imipramine and amitriptyline, has been found to potentiate their antidepressant action. Such a combination should, however, be regarded as experimental at present and should be undertaken only with considerable caution.

Once a patient has responded well to ECT or to a tricyclic antidepressant he should be maintained on a lower dose of tricyclic drug for some six months after recovery in order to minimise the risk of relapse.

2 *Monoamine oxidase inhibitors (MAOI)* From the evidence provided from well-controlled clinical trials it would appear that MAOI are not as effective as the tricyclic antidepressants in depressive illness. In addition they have the serious disadvantages of producing hypertensive reactions with certain foods, interacting with drugs like pethidine and causing liver damage. Occasionally, however, they can produce remissions in patients where all else has failed. The available drugs in this group are listed in Table 5. Particular caution should be maintained when changing from a MAOI to a tricyclic antidepressant or vice versa. It is safest to allow a two week drug-free interval between the two.

L-tryptophan, the amino-acid precursor of 5HT, in a dose of 5–9 g per day, has been reported to increase the efficacy of MAOI in depression, possibly by increasing the availability of 5HT at the synaptic junction. Furthermore, claims have been made that l-tryptophan alone is equally effective; certain workers have gone so far as to say that l-trytophan is as effective as ECT. These latter claims have not been substantiated however.

3 *Neuroleptic drugs* Certain neuroleptic compounds have been used in depressive illness. While some studies have revealed that chlorpromazine (Largactil, Thorazine) and flupenthixol (Fluanxol) are useful in the treatment of depressive illness, most authorities would recommend starting treatment with a tricyclic drug rather than a neuroleptic, as more recent trials have shown their clear superiority.

4 *Lithium* Lithium was originally introduced as a treatment for mania but some workers have claimed that it is also effective in certain cases of depressive illness (particularly 'bipolar' depression). In general, however, lithium is not as effective as the tricyclic compounds in depressive illness.

Depressive reactions (reactive depression, neurotic depression)

As we have already indicated, depressive reactions, in contrast to depressive illness, respond more readily to anxiolytic sedatives than to antidepressants, although those antidepressant drugs with a pronounced sedative action, such as amitriptyline and doxepin, may be effective. They are especially useful when it is uncertain which type of depression is present.

The choice of the appropriate anxiolytic sedative to use in this condition lies largely among the benzodiazepine groups of drugs (see chapter 7). In addition counselling and supportive psychotherapy should form an integral part of the treatment programme.

Mania

1 *Neuroleptic drugs* The manic patient, with his non-stop activity, constant pressure of talk, bellicose self-confidence and inability to focus on any activity for more than a moment, will nearly always require urgent treatment, preferably in hospital. The neuroleptic drugs (see chapter 5), particularly the phenothiazine compound chlorpromazine (Largactil, Thorazine) and the butyrophenone, haloperidol (Serenace, Haldol) have proved to be very effective in the emergency treatment of mania.

Initially, if the patient is unwilling to take oral medication, intramuscular administration of some 250–500 mg chlorpromazine or 3–10 mg haloperidol will be required. This may need to be repeated until the patient becomes sufficiently cooperative to take the drug orally. It is usually a matter of trial and error to determine the dose which is adequate to control the symptoms without being too sedating. For chlorpromazine it is likely to lie between 75 and 200 mg three times daily and for haloperidol to be between 1·5 mg and 6 mg twice daily. Such high doses of neuroleptics may produce marked parkinsonian effects which can be alleviated by antiparkinsonian drugs such as benzhexol (Artane) 2–4 mg three times daily, or orphenadrine (Disipal) 50–100 mg three times daily (see chapter 5).

Medication should be continued for several weeks after the patient has returned to normal, when it can be cautiously reduced. However, should any of the signs of mania reappear, treatment will then need to be maintained at a higher dose for another period of several weeks.

2 *Lithium* Although lithium was introduced as an effective treatment for mania as early as 1949, by Cade in Australia, it was used very little until the late 1960s. It would appear from well-controlled trials that lithium carbonate has a definite therapeutic effect in mania, but this effect usually takes about a week to appear. As there is such a relatively long delay in onset of action, lithium is not particularly useful as the sole initial treatment in mania because of the need for a drug with a much more rapid action (see above). It can, however, be given at the same time as a neuroleptic, and the neuroleptic can then be gradually tailed off as the lithium takes effect.

When administering lithium carbonate, either as the standard tablet (Camcolit) or as the longer acting preparation (Priadel) it is essential to ensure that the plasma levels remain below 1·5 milli-equivalents per litre. Above this level toxic effects appear, and above 2 mEq/L these toxic effects can prove extremely dangerous (see below). On the other hand, in order to ensure that an effective dose is being given, it is advisable to maintain the plasma level of lithium above 0·6 mEq/L. Thus the safe but effective range of plasma lithium levels is 0·6–1·5 mEq/L. It is necessary to monitor plasma levels frequently (at least weekly) for the first few weeks of treatment.

Once the appropriate dose has been established to maintain adequate plasma levels then blood level estimations need only be repeated monthly unless the patient develops an intercurrent illness.

Early signs of toxicity include a fine tremor of the hands and a sensation of nausea or abdominal discomfort. If the plasma level of lithium rises further it can lead to drowsiness, vomiting and diarrhoea; at this point lithium should be stopped immediately and the blood level measured as a matter of urgency. If this is not done the clinical state may deteriorate further with coma and death ensuing. With severe lithium poisoning haemodialysis may be necessary. Under no circumstances should lithium be administered to a patient with a history of serious renal or cardiac disease, and it should only be given with great circumspection to a patient with hypothyroidism, as lithium interferes with thyroid metabolism, and can produce frank myxoedema.

3 *5HT Antagonists* As a result of experimental work in the young chick, Dewhurst suggested that the clinical condition of mania may be the consequence of a raised level of 5-hydroxy-tryptamine within the central nervous system. He went on to reason that if this were the case then a specific inhibitor of 5HT should prove an effective and rational treatment for mania. Methysergide is one such specific 5HT antagonist. Early uncontrolled reports of methysergide (6–8 mg daily) in mania were enthusiastic, but these claims for its efficacy were not substantiated by carefully-controlled trials. It would appear that, in spite of the theoretical attractions, methysergide is not likely to be generally useful in the management of mania. Fenfluramine, a potent appetite suppressant (see chapter 12), is also reported to have anti-5HT properties. It is of some potential significance, therefore, that fenfluramine has been reported as being effective in mania.

Prophylaxis of affective disorders

Many patients who have a depressive illness or an attack of mania give a history of previous episodes of either mania or depression. These periods of illness tend to become more frequent with time, eventually occurring once or twice a year. It would obviously be of considerable benefit to such patients if these attacks of affective disorder could be prevented. Schou and his colleagues in Denmark have presented convincing evidence that continuous administration of lithium carbonate (maintaining a plasma level of between 0·6 and 1·5 mEq/L) significantly reduces the relapse rate. These Danish findings have now been confirmed by other investigators. Therefore patients with recurrent attacks of depressive illness (*not* depressive reactions or neurotic depression) and mania should be given a trial of lithium prophylaxis. The dosage required to maintain adequate blood levels will be similar to that used in the treatment of mania (see above), i.e. 0·6 to 1·5 g per day. Any signs of toxicity (see above) should be an indication for checking the serum level, and if necessary stopping the drug for a few days. As before, no patients with serious cardiac or renal disease should be treated with lithium and care must be taken in cases where there is any suggestion of hypothyroidism. With these provisos, suitable patients may be safely and successfully maintained on lithium medication for years.

Table 5 *Antidepressant drugs*

Approved name	Proprietary name	Recommended dose (daily unless stated otherwise)	Remarks
Tricyclic anti-depressants			
imipramine	Tofranil	75–200 mg	The 'standard' tricyclic compound against which others are compared. Autonomic and cardiac effects may be pronounced at higher dosage. Takes 10–14 days to act
desipramine	Pertofran Norpramine	75–200 mg	The demethylated metabolite of imipramine; no advantages over imipramine
trimipramine	Surmontil	50–100 mg (as single dose before retiring)	Methylated derivative of imipramine; no obvious advantages over other tricyclics
clomipramine	Anafranil	50–150 mg (can be given as infusion)	Chloro-derivative of imipramine; no obvious advantages over imipramine. Can be given by intravenous infusion. Said to be useful in obsessional and phobic disorders
amitriptyline	Tryptizol Elavil	75–200 mg	Effective antidepressant with sedative properties, particularly useful in depressive illness accompanied by anxiety. Takes 10–14 days to act fully
	Lentizol	50–100 mg sustained release tablets at night	

Table 5—*Contd.*

Approved name	Proprietary name	Recommended dose (daily unless stated otherwise)	Remarks
nortriptyline	Aventyl	75–200 mg	Demethylated derivative of amitriptyline; no obvious advantage over amitriptyline
protriptyline	Condordin Triptil Vivactil	15–60 mg	Unsaturated analogue of nortriptyline; the most rapidly acting of the tricyclics. Effective within 5–10 days
doxepin	Sinequan	75–150 mg	Oxepin derivative of amitriptyline. Pronounced anxiolytic effect. Antidepressant activity equal to imipramine and amitriptyline
dothiepin	Prothiaden	75–150 mg	Thiapin derivative of amitriptyline. As effective as amitriptyline with fewer autonomic side-effects
iprindole	Prondol	45–90 mg	An indole central ring with imipramine side-chain. As effective as imipramine and amitriptyline with fewer autonomic effects. May cause liver damage
opipramol	Insidon Ensidon	100–150 mg	Imipramine nucleus with piperazine side-chain. No advantage over imipramine
dibenzepin	Noveril	240–480 mg	Structure resembles imipramine with side-chain in different position. Clinically equivalent to imipramine

Table 5—*Contd.*

Approved name	Proprietary name	Recommended dose (daily unless stated otherwise)	Remarks
Monoamine oxidase inhibitors			Little convincing evidence of efficacy in depressive illness, although certain patients respond well. All MAOI can cause severe hypertensive reaction with tyramine-containing foods (e.g. cheese), sympatho-mimetic amines and tricyclic antidepressants. Also potentiate action of pethidine and alcohol.
1 *hydrazines*			
phenelzine	Nardil	30–90 mg	
isocarboxazid	Marplan	20–40 mg	
nialamide	Niamid	50–150 mg	
mebanazine	Actomol	5–30 mg	
iproniazid	Marsilid	50–75 mg	
2 *non-hydrazines*			
tranyl-cypromine	Parnate	20–40 mg	May cause liver damage. Of some value in management of phobic disorders. Maybe genetically determined slow acetylators respond best to phenelzine due to reduced rate of metabolism of the drug.

Suggestions for further reading

ASHCROFT, G. W., 'Modified amine hypothesis for the aetiology of affective illness', *Lancet*, Vol. 2, pp. 573–7, 1972.

COPPEN, A., and WALK, A., *Recent Developments in Affective Disorders*, *British Journal of Psychiatry*, Special Publication, No. 2, 1968.

GERSHON, S., 'Lithium in mania', *Clinical Pharmacology and Therapeutics*. Vol. 11, pp. 168–87, 1970.

KLERMAN, G. L., and PAYKEL, E., 'The tricyclic antidepressants', *Principles of Psychopharmacology*, W. G. Clarke and J. del Guidice (eds), Academic Press, New York, 1970.

SCHILDKARUT, J. J., 'Catecholamine metabolism and affective illnesses', *Biochemistry, Schizophrenias and Affective Illnesses*, H. E. Himwich (ed.), Williams & Wilkins, Baltimore, 1970.

SCHOU, M., ANDISEN, A., and BAASTRUP, P. C., 'The practical management of lithium treatment', *British Journal of Hospital Medicine*, Vol. 6, pp. 53–6, 1971.

Anxiety 7

Anxiety is an inevitable by-product of the process by which a person learns to become a member of society . . . . The fact that the human being can experience fear permits this learning to take place. In the process anxiety arises.   *Levitt*

Psychophysiology of anxiety

Anxiety and fear play a vital role in all human societies. To feel anxious in the face of a threatening stimulus is both normal and appropriate; it is only when the anxiety becomes so severe as to be incapacitating, or arises without reasonable cause, that clinical intervention is indicated. Unfortunately this occurs all too frequently. In a large epidemiological survey in the London area it was found that 14 per cent of the population at risk consulted the doctor at least once during the course of a year for symptoms which were a reflection of underlying anxiety. A Scandinavian study revealed that one-third of the adult population had overt symptoms of anxiety, nervousness or tension; 5 per cent had symptoms severe enough to warrant the diagnosis of an anxiety state.

The subjective awareness of anxiety and fear is associated with general 'arousal' of the central nervous system plus peripheral autonomic discharge. Stimuli which are seen as threatening produce activation of the reticular activating system (RAS) in the brain stem, probably via corticofugal pathways passing down from the cerebral cortex to the reticular formation, the cortex classifying the particular stimuli as being threatening or not. It is likely that the cerebral cortex and the RAS together constitute a feedback-control system maintaining an optimal arousal level. Through this system when cortical activity is great the RAS activity is inhibited, thereby preventing too great an arousal level. Should this inhibition of the RAS break down then the cortical activity may continue unchecked, leading to a state of incapacitating anxiety.

In addition other areas of the brain are clearly involved in the pathogenesis of anxiety, particularly the structures grouped in the limbic system, including the amygdala and the hippocampus, together with areas in the hypothalamus. Stimulation of the posterior hypothalamus in laboratory animals leads to behaviour suggestive of a panic reaction; stimulation of the same area in humans is reported as being most unpleasant. It is believed that the hypothalamic centres, which probably regulate the autonomic discharge seen in anxiety, are themselves under the control of the hippocampus and amygdala; on the one hand the amygdala increases, and on the other the hippocampus and septal region inhibits the hypothalamic response to threatening stimuli.

It has been found that stimulation of the centro-medial hypothalamus in a normally placid cat will generate aggressive behaviour which can be considerably modified by simultaneous stimulation of the amygdala. Furthermore, such electrical stimulation of the amygdala produces a rapid rise in 17-hydroxycortico steroids presumably by increasing ACTH production via the hypothalamic pituitary axis.

Additional experimental evidence for the view that these regions of the brain are important in the production of anxiety comes from studies using implanted electrodes. When electrodes are placed in certain areas of the brain of a rat (e.g. the septal region and the lateral hypothalamus), and the animal can turn on the current by pressing a lever with its foot (self-stimulation), it is repeatedly found that the rat will continuously stimulate itself in this way for hours at a time, ignoring food and water. If an animal has been trained to expect a shock on hearing a click it will normally cower in a corner of its cage when the click sounds. If however it is able to self-stimulate its septal area it will ignore the sound of the click and even when the electric shock is applied to its feet it will not show any sign of a fear reaction; it just keeps on self-stimulating.

The hippocampal–amygdala system is in turn regulated by the cerebral cortex which, as we have seen, is modulated by the RAS through a feedback loop.

Histochemical studies have shown that the neurones of the lower brain stem, where the RAS is situated, contain noradrenaline (NA) and dopamine (DA). These particular neurones have widespread synaptic connections with the limbic system and it has been postulated that NA may act as the transmitter in the system underlying anxiety responses, particularly as the NA levels in NA cells rise during the performance of a conditioned avoidance response. In addition to the NA cells in the lower brain stem there are others projecting to the lateral hypothalamus and the hippocampus which synthesise 5-hydroxytryptamine (5HT). It could be that these two cell types themselves act reciprocally, the NA cell system increasing the anxiety response and the 5HT cell system reducing it. In keeping with this hypothesis is the finding that members of the benzodiazepine group of drugs (see below) which are effective in the treatment of anxiety, can increase brain 5HT levels.

Whatever the central mechanism involved, the subjective experience of anxiety is usually accompanied by widespread sympathetic discharge together with a steep rise in circulating catecholamines. The particular autonomic changes which have been most studied are those occurring in the cardiovascular system and those in the palmar sweat glands.

Increased anxiety has long been known to be associated with a quickening of the heart. Measurements of peripheral blood flow, using venous occlusion plethysmography, have demonstrated that when an individual is anxious his forearm blood flow also increases. These autonomic responses can reinforce the central awareness of anxiety and thus compound the severity of the symptoms; such cardiovascular concomitants frequently cause the patient to seek medical advice.

The palmar sweat glands, which have little thermoregulatory function, are innervated by the sympathetic nervous system but, unlike the rest of this system, are cholinergic rather than adrenergic. Thus drugs blocking adrenergic responses (i.e. the beta-adrenergic blockers—see below) do not affect increased palmar sweating although they can effectively reduce psychogenic tachycardia. The level of palmar sweating determines the electrical resistance of the palmar skin. When sweating is marked, resistance is low, and vice versa. This phenomenon is the basis of the so-called psychogalvanic response (see chapter 3) which has proved to be a most useful physiological variable with which to compare states of psychological arousal.

The autonomic accompaniments of anxiety are so pervasive that at one time it was thought that they, rather than any central phenomena, actually caused the anxiety. This view was shown to be erroneous by Cannon and it came to be accepted that the experience of anxiety was entirely dependent on the central state, with little reference to what was occurring peripherally.

This was too great a swing of the pendulum, as Schachter showed. In a series of ingenious experiments he revealed that it is the *interaction* between peripheral autonomic events and the central nervous system which determine the specific emotional response observed in a particular situation. When normal subjects received injections of adrenaline and were told what to expect (i.e. tachycardia, etc.) they did not experience marked emotions even in the face of provocation, whereas those subjects who were not informed what to expect in the way of physiological changes reacted much more vigorously to amusing situations as well as to threatening ones. Schachter concluded that the autonomic events increase central arousal, but the way the individual behaves when aroused is determined by what is happening around him. If he is in a threatening situation he becomes angry or fearful, whereas if he is in an amusing situation he becomes happy. In summary, the direction of the emotion experienced is determined by the nature of the situation and the personality of the individual, while the amplitude of the emotional response is modified by the degree of autonomic discharge.

More recently there have been investigations into possible metabolic mechanisms underlying anxiety. It had been noted that certain individuals became particularly anxious after vigorous exercise, and the suggestion was made that such an exacerbation of anxiety might be due to the increase in circulating lactate which occurs under such conditions. Pitts and McClure examined this possibility by infusing a half-molar lactate solution into patients who had no panic attacks, as well as into normal controls, and comparing the findings with those occurring after infusion of isoosmotic glucose solutions and lactate plus added calcium. Their findings were clear cut: the great majority of the patients with a history of panic attacks developed similar attacks when receiving a lactate infusion, but not a glucose infusion. Only a small proportion of the normal controls responded in this way. Addition of calcium appeared to modify the lactate response in the patients. On the basis of their findings Pitts and McClure suggested that anxiety symptoms have 'a common determining biochemical mechanism involving the complexing of ionized calcium'. They assumed that the experience of anxiety was associated with an increase in circulating catecholamines which in turn led to a rise in the serum lactate levels which interfered with neural transmission by interacting with calcium at the neuronal membrane.

More recently doubt has been cast on this hypothesis by the observations that anxiety can occur without increased circulating lactate, and that increased lactate does not necessarily lead to anxiety. Furthermore, the tachycardia accompanying lactate infusion is not affected by beta-adrenergic blockade, whereas psychogenic tachycardia is. The counter-suggestion has been made that the effects noted with lactate infusions are due primarily to a metabolic alkalosis with a rising blood bicarbonate level, not to interference with calcium binding by the lactate ions.

While the original observation that lactate infusion can cause severe anxiety attacks in predisposed individuals has been confirmed in a number of centres, both the underlying explanation and the clinical relevance of these findings remain uncertain.

Pharmacology of anxiolytic-sedative drugs

Drugs used in the treatment of anxiety states may be divided broadly into two groups, namely those which act primarily on the central nervous system and those which block peripheral autonomic receptors.

Centrally acting drugs

These are known as anxiolytic sedatives (sometimes referred to as minor tranquillisers). There is as yet no purely anxiolytic compound, all have some sedative properties.

1 *Barbiturate drugs* Although the most important use of the barbiturates is as hypnotics to induce sleep they are effective anxiolytic sedatives in small doses. Phenobarbitone and amylobarbitone are the most commonly used barbiturates for this purpose. While their mode of action is not clearly understood, they are known to produce widespread depression of neuronal activity throughout the brain, particularly in synapses of the reticular activating system in the brain stem. At the molecular level, the barbiturate drugs probably act by depressing formation of high energy phosphate which is essential for normal brain activity.

The ratio between the dose of a barbiturate drug, such as phenobarbitone, necessary to relieve symptoms and signs of anxiety and that which produces other evidence of central nervous depression is small. For this reason it is difficult to obtain a satisfactory anxiolytic effect without some reduction of alertness and vigilance. In some cases this may lead to marked impairment of consciousness and sleep. As the dose is increased central nervous depression becomes still more marked with the involvement of respiratory and vasomotor centres.

Apart from the dangers of overdosage, there are two other important disadvantages which barbiturates possess:

(i) a tendency to produce drug dependence
(ii) induction of liver microsomal enzymes.

Therapeutic doses of barbiturate drugs are sufficient to stimulate the activity of liver microsomal enzyme systems concerned with their own metabolism and with that of other drugs. This stimulating effect, or induction, is associated with increased liver weight, increased production of microsomal protein, and changes in the smooth membrane of the endoplasmic reticulum. Among the drugs whose half-lives are known to be reduced by treatment with barbiturate drugs are: (i) coumarin anticoagulants, leading to a reduction in their hypoprothrombinaemic effects (ii) phenytoin, reducing its anticonvulsant effect (iii) griseofulvin, the antifungal agent and (iv) amidopyrine.

The most important of these interactions is with the coumarin drugs. It is not uncommon for a patient admitted to hospital following a myocardial infarction to be treated with a coumarin anticoagulant drug and also with a barbiturate such as phenobarbitone to relieve anxiety and mental distress. The latter drug, by liver enzyme induction, increases the rate of hydroxylation of the coumarin drug so reducing its anticoagulant effect, which leads in turn to an increase in the dose required to obtain the desired prolongation of prothrombin time. When the barbiturate drug is withdrawn, often when the patient leaves hospital, the microsomal enzyme activity returns to normal over a period of two or three weeks. Unless the dose of the anticoagulant drug is reduced during this period, a dangerous increase in prothrombin time may occur as its rate of metabolism returns to normal, producing a potentially dangerous haemorrhagic tendency.

Whenever a barbiturate drug is prescribed, particularly on a long-term basis, its possible interaction with other substances should be considered. Little is known of the significance or extent of enzyme induction in man, but its importance is probably much greater than has been realised.

2 *Benzodiazepine drugs* These drugs have been introduced into clinical medicine relatively recently, but have already established themselves as a major advance in the treatment of anxiety states. When given to animals in small doses they appear to act primarily on subcortical structures such as the amygdala and hippocampus of the limbic system, without affecting the cerebral cortex. It has been suggested, on the basis of animal experiments, that they act by increasing the level of available 5HT in these centres. Clinically, the benzodiazepine drugs have an anxiolytic action in doses which do not produce sedation, although higher doses may cause drowsiness and lethargy. Physical as well as psychological dependence to these drugs has been described and convulsions have occurred when they have been withdrawn following protracted administration in high doses.

Overdosage with these agents, accidentally or for suicidal purposes, produces drowsiness, sleep, inco-ordination, muscle weakness, ataxia and dysarthria. In a large series of cases of chlordiazepoxide intoxication in which the dose ingested ranged from 60 to 100 mg the patients were at no time completely unrousable. Although relatively safe when taken alone, benzodiazepines may potentiate the central depressant effects of alcohol and barbiturate drugs and such combinations can be dangerous.

There are several benzodiazepine drugs available for the treatment of anxiety. The most commonly used are:

(i) chlordiazepoxide (Librium), an effective tranquillising drug used in doses of 10–100 mg daily; 10 mg is approximately equivalent to 75 mg amylobarbitone;
(ii) diazepam (Valium), probably a more effective anxiolytic, but also produces more drowsiness and euphoria than chlordiazepoxide. Doses vary from 5–50 mg daily. It may be used intravenously to control fits in status epilepticus, and in premedication for surgery and cardioversion;
(iii) medazepam (Nobrium);
(iv) oxazepam (Serenid), is a metabolite of diazepam;
(v) lorazepam (Ativan), a derivative of oxazepam;
(vi) clorazepate (Tranxene), can be given once daily.

Other members of this group of compounds, nitrazepam (Mogadon) and flurazepam (Dalmane) are used as hypnotics (see chapter 10).

3 *Propanediols* Meprobamate, like mephenesin from which it is derived, is a skeletal muscle-relaxing compound in experimental animals, but in addition has tranquillising properties in man. It appears that its principle mechanism of action as an anxiolytic agent is to block activity between the cerebral cortex and subcortical structures, thus interfering with centrally mediated autonomic responses. In doses of about 400 mg little if any sedation occurs, but 800 mg or more has marked hypnotic properties in many patients. Several controlled trials have shown that meprobamate is superior to barbiturates as a hypnotic agent, probably because of its relative lack of hang-over effects.

Habituation occurs to meprobamate, and abstinence symptoms and epileptiform convulsions on withdrawal of the drug have been reported. Overdosage produces pronounced central nervous depression with somnolence and hypotonia, and finally coma.

Although meprobamate is widely prescribed in musculoskeletal disorders it is unlikely to be effective in reducing muscle spasm except where the spasm is due to an underlying anxiety state.

4 *Diphenylamines* The two drugs in this group, hydroxyzine and benactyzine, have now largely been superseded.

5 *Neuroleptics* ('major tranquillisers') (see chapter 5)

(i) *Chlorpromazine* (Largactil, Thorazine) This drug is not as effective in the treatment of anxiety as amylobarbitone.

(ii) *Trifluoperazine* (Stelazine) Several well-controlled studies have indicated that trifluoperazine is of some use in anxiety as well as in schizophrenia, but it would seem to possess no advantages over the barbiturates or benzodiazepines in this situation.

(iii) *Haloperidol* (Serenace) This drug has recently been promoted for use in anxiety. Again no particular advantage over the standard compound is apparent.

(iv) *Oxypertine* (Integrin) In contrast to the other neuroleptics this drug may have a definite place in the management of anxiety. In one study, 10 mg three times daily was found to be more effective than diazepam 5 mg three times daily, with less psychomotor disturbance; other trials however have failed to reveal any such superiority of oxypertine over diazepam.

(v) *Pimozide* (Orap) This is a member of the longer acting diphenylbutylpiperidine group of compounds. Pimozide only needs to be given once daily in a dose of 2–4 mg. Preliminary trials indicate that when given in this way it is virtually equal in efficacy to chlordiazepoxide.

6 *Other compounds: benzoctamine* (Tacitin). A molecule with an unusual steric structure, it possesses both anxiolytic and muscle relaxant properties. Its place in the management of anxiety is uncertain as yet.

A wide variety of other centrally acting drugs have at one time or another been tried in the treatment of anxiety symptoms. While many have been shown under double-blind conditions to be more effective than placebo, few, if any, are clearly better than barbiturates or benzodiazepines (see Table 6).

The sedative action of alcohol should not be forgotten in transient or mild anxiety states, particularly in elderly patients. Insomnia, restlessness and nervousness may often be allayed by the judicious use of an alcoholic beverage.

Peripherally acting drugs

Many of the manifestations of anxiety already described are probably due to an increased release of adrenaline and noradrenaline from the adrenal medulla and sympathetic nerves, and changes in urinary excretion of these amines and their metabolites have been demonstrated in patients suffering from anxiety. For this reason adrenergic blockade with drugs, such as propranolol, is effective in reducing or abolishing anxiety symptoms, particularly those which are predominantly autonomic in nature like palpitations and tremor. Relatively small doses of propranolol such as 10 or 20 mg six- or eight-hourly may be used together with small doses of a barbiturate or benzodiazepine drug. It must be remembered that, in some patients, bronchial asthma is a manifestation of anxiety; when this happens propranolol and other beta blockers are contra-indicated.

Drug treatment of anxiety

Mild to moderate anxiety symptoms

When a patient presents with either the psychological symptoms of anxiety (excessive worrying, inability to concentrate, difficulty in getting off to sleep) or its somatic accompaniments (palpitations, tension headaches, sweaty palms), the first step is to establish whether or not there is a reasonable cause for these symptoms to arise at that particular time. If so, it may be possible for the situation to be adjusted in such a way that the anxiety-provoking circumstances no longer apply.

Recognition of the underlying cause may, therefore, be itself of considerable therapeutic benefit. If, however, as is so often the case, the causative factors cannot be defined or modified, or there are no adequate grounds for the patient's symptoms, symptomatic relief with drugs together with psychological support is the next step. Before starting drug treatment it should be determined whether or not the patient's symptoms are but an acute episode in a normally non-anxious individual, or whether they reflect a long-standing predisposition to the development of frequent, perhaps even continuous, anxiety. In the former situation it is likely that remission will occur without any definitive therapeutic intervention. 40–50 per cent of such cases have been shown to remit spontaneously, although anxiolytic sedative drugs may increase this remission rate still further. In contrast, patients with chronic anxiety symptoms will more frequently require drug treatment, often for considerable periods of time, and at a dosage greater than patients with acute anxiety.

Of the available drugs the choice largely lies between a barbiturate or a benzodiazepine compound. The barbiturates have the inestimable advantage of being well-tested by time and are also the least expensive. They can, however, be dangerous if taken injudiciously and are perhaps more prone to produce drug dependence than the benzodiazepines. Recommended dosage varies from 50 mg two or three times a day in a case of mild anxiety to 100 mg three or four times a day in a more severe case. There is little to choose between one barbiturate and another.

The benzodiazepine compounds are as effective as the barbiturates and are certainly safer. However they are not without pronounced sedative effects and can produce marked ataxia. Whether one member of this group of drugs possesses any distinct advantages over the others is open to question. When comparisons have been made between them it has usually been on the basis of fixed dosages, so that the finding that diazepam 5 mg three times daily is more effective than chlordiazepoxide 10 mg three times daily does not necessarily imply that an increased dose of chlordiazepoxide would not be better still. Probably the benzodiazepine of first choice should be diazepam, with a dose ranging from 2 mg twice a day in a patient with mild symptoms, or in an elderly patient, to 20 mg three or four times a day in a patient with incapacitating anxiety (see below). Of the others, oxazepam (10 to 15 mg two to four times a day) would appear to possess some theoretical advantage over diazepam which is itself metabolised to oxazepam in the body.

When there is a pronounced cardiovascular element in the symptomatology, with one of the patient's main complaints being tachycardia, it may be helpful to prescribe a beta-adrenergic blocking compound in addition to the anxiolytic sedative. Propranolol 10 to 20 mg three or four times a day has been shown to be effective; other compounds in this group like practolol, oxprenolol and sotalol may also prove of value.

Severe anxiety state

When a patient presents with symptoms of anxiety so severe that he is incapable of functioning at all effectively either at work or at home it is necessary, whatever the cause and whatever the underlying personality, to reduce the level of central arousal as rapidly as possible. In extreme cases parenteral administration of an anxiolytic sedative may be initially required; either amylobarbitone sodium 300 mg intramuscularly or diazepam 10 mg intravenously. Subsequent large doses of oral medication should be prescribed for the first few days: amylobarbitone sodium 150 mg four times a day; or a benzodiazepine such as diazepam 15 to 20 mg four times daily; or oxazepam 15–30 mg three times daily. Additional sedation at night is usually needed (see chapter 10).

When the patient has been adequately sedated (and such a regime may well require hospitalisation) the dosage of drugs can be reduced gradually to a level where little or no daytime drowsiness is produced.

Some patients who present with an anxiety attack severe enough to warrant such measures may eventually be able to do without any medication, but most will require long-term administration of an anxiolytic sedative in the dosages recommended for mild to moderate anxiety.

Panic attacks

Certain individuals get attacks of overwhelming panic, often for no obvious reason. Such attacks may occur as frequently as twice a week or, on the other hand, be very occasional. The attacks are characterised by a subjective feeling of terror related to a sensation of imminent death, together with pronounced tremulousness, profuse sweating and marked tachycardia. They usually occur in a public place and not unnaturally cause considerable alarm in those witnessing the attack. In most cases an ambulance is called and the patient rushed to hospital, but by the time he or she gets there the attack has abated considerably. If not, parenteral amylobarbitone (300 mg intramuscularly) or diazepam (10 mg intravenously) should calm the patient adequately.

When the attack has settled, long-term medication will often help in reducing the frequency of attacks; this should be as recommended for cases of moderate anxiety. In many of the patients, the attack begins with tachycardia; this frightens the patient into believing he is about to have a 'heart attack' which in turn exacerbates the tachycardia and leads in time to greater fearfulness. Beta-adrenergic blocking drugs may reduce the tendency to tachycardia and thus reduce the likelihood of a full-blown panic attack.

It has been suggested that such panic attacks are associated with a considerable rise in the serum lactate concentration (see above), and that the accompanying autonomic changes are themselves secondary to the raised serum lactate level. If the patient can be taught to realise that such autonomic effects do not themselves presage immediate death, he should be able to tolerate the somatic symptoms with greater equanimity and without developing a panic attack. Such reasoning forms the theoretical basis for a new approach to the long-term management of patients with panic attacks. In this treatment, the lactate level is deliberately raised and the autonomic discharge is produced in a hospital setting in the presence of doctors. When the patient realises that nothing terrible does in fact happen he is able to tolerate the autonomic symptoms, as he has learned that they will not cause him any permanent harm. This approach can only be conducted in hospital and then under very carefully controlled conditions.

Situational anxiety and phobias

The term situational anxiety includes all the commonly recognised phobic symptoms. In addition, it includes those clinical states like psychogenic impotence and frigidity which are basically the result of anxiety confined to the sexual situation (see chapter 11). Phobias often arise as the result of a learned experience. Unfortunately the lesson is learned too well and the patient becomes unable to accept the fact that he is unlikely to come to any further harm in the particular situation. There would appear to be three main categories of phobias: (1) specific phobias—a fear of spiders, a fear of heights (2) social phobias—a fear of meeting people or of eating in public (3) agoraphobia—a general fear of being away from the security of one's home.

In recent years it has come to be accepted that the most effective therapeutic approach to such conditions is behaviour therapy. This 'specific desensitisation' may take the form of gradually reintroducing the patient, at first in imagination, later, in reality, to his feared situation. Another technique 'implosion' or 'flooding' is to plunge the patient in at the deep end, as it were, by repeatedly confronting him with his most feared object or getting him to imagine himself in his most feared situation. Opinions remain divided on the most effective of the two methods but it appears that the implosive technique is better for agoraphobes, the great majority of whom fail to respond to specific desensitisation, while specific desensitisation works best in patients with specific phobias.

In both these treatments, psychotropic drugs are useful in producing the required reduction of central arousal for the relearning to take place. They can be prescribed as a long-term measure, for which a barbiturate or a benzodiazepine is useful. In addition, the actual desensitisation or implosive procedure may be greatly facilitated by intravenous infusion of a rapidly metabolised barbiturate, methohexitone sodium (Brietal, Brevital) or a eugenol derivative, propanidid (Epontol) which is even more rapidly metabolised. These compounds are infused slowly intravenously during the course of a treatment session lasting up to thirty minutes. It is very important to avoid injecting too rapidly or the patient may be put to sleep. Furthermore it is absolutely necessary to have resuscitation apparatus at hand, together with a syringe charged with 1:1000 adrenaline before undertaking this treatment in case of an anaphylactoid reaction. Although both methohexitone and propanidid are equally effective, propanidid has the great practical advantage of causing less post-treatment drowsiness and a more rapid recovery. Even so, patients should be strongly discouraged from driving an automobile for several hours after a treatment session.

Apart from behaviour therapy, some recent studies have indicated that monoamine oxidase inhibitors, such as phenelzine (Nardil) 15 mg three times daily, may produce considerable improvement. While the rate of improvement with monoamine oxidase inhibition is quicker than with behaviour therapy, the tendency to relapse is much more marked with MAOI. As yet there have been few direct comparisons of MAOI with benzodiazepines in phobias; until such comparisons are undertaken, the exact place of MAOI in phobias must remain uncertain. Some authorities recommend gradually decreasing doses of benzodiazepines (beginning with intravenous diazepam in a 10 mg dose) together with gradual retraining; again whether or not this is better than MAOI treatment is undetermined.

Reports have recently appeared which indicate that intravenous infusion of the tricyclic antidepressant, clomipramine (Anafranil) may markedly ameliorate phobic symptoms. Until controlled trials have been performed these claims must be regarded as unconfirmed.

Table 6   *Anxiolytic drugs*

Approved name	Proprietary name	Recommended dose (*daily unless stated otherwise*)	Remarks
barbiturates			
amylobarbitone sodium (UK) amobarbitol (USA)	Sodium amytal	150–400 mg daily in divided doses or 1 hour before anxiety-provoking situation	Can lead to over-sedation. Over-dosage can be fatal; therefore use sparingly if any question of suicidal risk. Produces physical dependence, particularly in doses exceeding 1 g per day. Liver enzyme induction may occur
phenobarbitone (UK) phenobarbitol (USA)	Luminal	150–400 mg	

Table 6—*Contd.*

Approved name	Proprietary name	Recommended dose (daily unless stated otherwise)	Remarks
benzodiazepines			
chlordiazepoxide	Librium	10–100 mg	⎫ Effective anxiolytic compounds. Affect the limbic system before the cerebral cortex. Main advantage over barbiturates is in safety factor. Can produce dependence but less likely than barbiturates. Little to choose between individual members of this group
diazepam	Valium	4–80 mg	
oxazepam	Serenid-D Serax	20–90 mg	
medazepam	Nobrium	10–50 mg	
lorazepam	Ativan	3–10 mg	⎭
clorazepate	Tranxene	15 mg	Administer once a day
propanediols			
meprobamate	Miltown Equanil	400–2400 mg	Rather weak anxiolytics. Developed from muscle-relaxants
tybamate	Benvil Solacen	500–1000 mg	More effective and with shorter half-life than meprobamate. Little if any advantage over benzodiazepines
diphenylmethanes			
hydroxyzine	Atarax Vistaril	50–100 mg	Generally superseded by benzodiazepines
benactyzine	Suavitil		
neuroleptics			
chlorpromazine	Largactil Thorazine	50–100 mg	Not as effective as barbiturates in anxiety
trifluoperazine	Stelazine	4–10 mg	Better than placebo. Not evaluated against benzodiazepines. Possibility of parkinsonian symptoms

Table 6—*Contd.*

Approved name	*Proprietary name*	*Recommended dose (daily unless stated otherwise)*	*Remarks*
haloperidol	Serenace	1–2 mg	No obvious advantage over benzodiazepines
oxypertine	Integrin	30–40 mg	As effective as benzodiazepines with possibly less psychomotor disturbance
pimozide	Orap	2–4 mg	Equal to benzodiazepines in efficacy. Administration required only once daily
tricyclic compounds			
doxepin	Sinequan	20–150 mg	Anxiolytic as well as anti-depressant. As effective as low-dose benzodiazepines but greater likelihood of autonomic effects
opipramol	Insidon Ensidon	100–150 mg	Tricyclic with piperazine side-chain. As effective as low-dose benzodiazepines
clomipramine	Anafranil	50–250 mg (by slow intravenous infusion)	Said to be of value in obsessional and phobic conditions
dibenzobicyclo-octadienes			
benzoctamine	Tacitin	20–100 mg	Equal in efficiency to benzodiazepines with similar sedative side-effects

Table 6—*Contd.*

Approved name	Proprietary name	Recommended dose (*daily unless stated otherwise*)	Remarks
miscellaneous			
fenfluramine	Ponderax	40–120 mg	Centrally sedating appetite suppressant of possible use in anxiety—particularly anxious obese patients
phenytoin (UK) diphenyl-hydantoin (USA)	Epanutin Dilantin	300 mg	Anticonvulsant shown to possess anxiolytic properties

Suggestions for further reading

BLACK, A. A., 'Drug treatment of anxiety', *British Journal of Hospital Medicine*, Vol. 2, pp. 1453–8, 1969.

LADER, M. H., and MARKS, I., *Clinical Anxiety*, Heinemann, London, 1971.

LADER, M. H., and WING, L., *Physiological Measures, Sedative Drugs and Morbid Anxiety*, Oxford University Press, London, 1966.

GUIRGEA, C., 'Pharmacological criteria for the classification of tranquillisers', *The Present Status of Psychotropic Drugs*, A. Cerletti and F. J. Bové (eds), *Excerpta Medica*, Amsterdam, 1969.

8 Organic psychiatric syndromes

The term 'organic psychiatric syndromes' refers to those conditions in which there is a disturbance of psychological function due to a definite physical cause. That is not to say that other psychiatric conditions, such as schizophrenia or mania, are not primarily due to physical causes; they may well be. It is just that we have not yet determined with any confidence what they are (see chapters 5 and 6). In the case of the organic psychiatric syndromes, the disruption of cerebral function leading to the psychological disturbance may either be temporary (acute) or permanent (chronic).

Such phenomena as metabolic upsets, anoxia, hypoglycaemia, high fever and acute poisons frequently produce an impairment of cerebral function with an accompanying disturbance of consciousness. This gives rise to the clinical condition known as an 'acute confusional state'. Usually improvement of the underlying cause is followed promptly by amelioration of the mental state. In contrast, where the psychological impairment is due to permanent damage of the brain, as in *dementia* and the *dysmnesic syndrome* (see below), no significant spontaneous improvement can be expected.

Acute confusional state (delirium)

Whenever the level of consciousness is impaired, however slightly, there is an associated reduction in attention, with an increase in distractability. The more profound the reduction in consciousness the greater the psychological disturbance. This lessening of attention leads to a failure in grasping instructions and in registering new information. The patient thus becomes seemingly un-cooperative, even truculent. In addition there may be delusions of persecution, and these, together with the restlessness and irritability which commonly occur, can make nursing difficult. Inability to register new information leads to disorientation in time and space. Such disorientation together with clouding of consciousness are cardinal features of an acute confusional state.

Other symptoms include hallucinations, particularly visual hallucinations, dysphasia and perseveration, disconnected thinking; anxiety, sometimes amounting to frank terror, can also be present, particularly in delirium tremens (see below).

An acute confusional state can be caused by a wide variety of conditions; anything which interferes with brain function can bring it about. However, the clinical picture is largely the same whatever the pathogenesis; it is determined not so much by the primary cause as by: (i) the intensity and duration of the cerebral disturbance (ii) the environmental stimuli present during the cerebral disturbance (iii) the previous personality and experience of the patient.

Treatment must first be directed towards the underlying cause, and in many cases this will be sufficient to improve the psychological state. When rapid improvement of the basic disturbance is not possible, and the behaviour of the patient remains disturbed, then additional treatment specifically directed towards improving the mental state is usually indicated. In most cases cautious medication with chlorpromazine (Largactil, Thorazine) (see chapter 5) will suffice. As cerebral function is already impaired, and a lowered blood pressure accompanies many of the conditions producing an acute confusional state, it is essential to start treatment with a relatively small dose: 25–50 mg either orally or intramuscularly. If this does not produce the desired effect, and provided that there has been no worsening of the patient's clinical condition, the drug can be given subsequently in a larger dose: 50–100 mg. Occasionally it may be necessary to exceed 150 mg but this must be done with great care as most patients with an acute confusional state are already physically ill; adding what amounts to yet another toxic substance may well not improve matters overall.

In patients with liver failure the impaired detoxication of many anxiolytic sedatives and narcotics leads to an exaggeration and prolongation of their pharmacological effects; thus great caution must be exercised.

Delirium tremens

In contrast to other toxic confusional states, delirium tremens arises as a result of withdrawal of a drug (alcohol) rather than its administration. In order to reduce these withdrawal symptoms, which are very alarming and can even prove fatal, it is advisable to prescribe a barbiturate, paraldehyde, one of the benzodiazepine group of drugs, or chlormethiazole. Relatively large doses, given either orally or systemically are usually required for adequate sedation: chlordiazepoxide (Librium) 25–50 mg, diazepam (Valium) 20–40 mg or chlormethiazole (Heminevrin) 1·5–2 g are probably the drugs of choice (even larger doses than this may be needed in resistant cases). Some authorities still recommend intramuscular paraldehyde: 10–12 mg to start with, increasing up to 40 mg if necessary. In addition many patients are dehydrated and require rapid measures to correct their fluid balance. Finally, chronic alcoholism is often accompanied by a relative deficiency of thiamine and other B vitamins. Because of this, large doses of B vitamins are usually given systemically to patients with delirium tremens.

Dementia

Dementia, a condition characterised by a waning of intellectual powers, impairment of memory (particularly the retention of new information), emotional lability, a coarsening of the personality together with increasing disinterest in personal appearance and hygiene, comes about as a result of degeneration or destruction of the cerebral cortex. This may be caused by a variety of conditions, including hereditary degenerative diseases, the so-called pre-senile dementias (Huntington's chorea, Pick's disease, Alzheimer's disease, Creutzfeld–Jacob's disease), trauma, toxic substances (lead and mercury), metabolic disturbance (prolonged hypo-glycaemia, myxoedema), pernicious anaemia, infections (particularly syphilis), and neoplasms. However, more common than any of the above are cerebral arteriosclerosis and 'senile' degeneration, both occurring much more frequently in the elderly. Recent surveys have revealed that of those aged sixty-five or over about 5 per cent are suffering from frank dementia and another 5 per cent are suffering from a milder form. The great majority in both categories are living in the community, institutional care being provided for relatively few. Approximately half of these individuals are suffering from cerebral degeneration secondary to arteriosclerosis; the other half have senile dementia.

Arteriosclerotic dementia

Dementia due to cerebral arteriosclerosis tends to run a fluctuating course. In addition, there are usually focal neurological signs together with a raised blood pressure. Post-mortem studies reveal widespread areas of cerebral softening. The greater the degree of intellectual impairment present the greater the total area of cerebral softening found. Unfortunately, treatment of established arteriosclerosis is largely unavailing; certainly by the time dementia has occurred no measures designed to alter such factors as the general blood pressure level are likely to do much good. However, some claims have been made for cyclandelate (Cyclospasmol), isoxsuprine (Duvadilan) and dihydroergotoxine (Hydergine) which appear to increase cerebral blood flow; improvement in intellectual capacity and memory has been reported after a few months continuous treatment with cyclandelate 400 mg four times daily. Unfortunately, there appeared to be no correlation between the degree of improvement in cerebral circulation observed with radio-circulograms and the level of improvement in psychometric test scores. Furthermore, the ward nursing staff failed to note any greater improvement in the patients given cyclandelate as compared to those given placebo. A more recently introduced compound naftidrofuryl (Praxiline) has been the subject of two small controlled trials. In both it proved superior to placebo. However, until more comprehensive studies have been completed, the place of these drugs in the treatment of arteriosclerotic dementia must remain uncertain. Treatment of associated disturbed behaviour is as for senile dementia (see below).

Senile dementia

In many respects senile dementia can be seen as a gross exaggeration of the normal ageing process, although whether the two differ qualitatively as well as quantitatively is an open question. From the pathological point of view, they would appear to differ only in degree, rather than kind. Normal ageing is associated with the appearance of so-called senile plaques (argentophil plaques) in the cerebral cortex. In senile dementia there are many more such plaques, and the greater the number of plaques the more severe the dementia. In contrast to arteriosclerotic dementia, the course is continuous and there are few, if any, focal neurological signs. There may be a family history of senile dementia, and it is this genetic predisposition which leads some authorities to consider that senile dementia is distinct from normal ageing.

Neurophysiologically there is often a slowing in the frequency and in the amount of the alpha rhythm in the EEG. There is also a slowing of conduction time in peripheral nerves, as well as a significant increase in latency in the EEG-recorded somatosensory evoked response. These findings suggest that the basic disturbance in senile dementia may be a generalised slowing of conduction within the nervous system.

There is no known treatment which effectively reverses or even halts the underlying pathological process. Controlled trials of a wide variety of substances including folic acid, androgenic hormones and procaine hydrochloride (substance 'H') have shown them all to be quite ineffective. Many patients, particularly in the later stages of the disease, exhibit disturbed behaviour both during the day and in the night. The most suitable drug for daytime control is thioridazine (Melleril) in a dose of 25–100 mg given up to three times daily. While extrapyramidal symtoms are less likely with this drug than with other phenothiazine compounds, there is a risk of retrolental fibroplasia and of retinitis if a daily dosage of 600 mg is continued for more than a few months. A suitable alternative drug is chlorpromazine given in the same dosage, but here the risk of extrapyramidal reactions is greater.

For night sedation chloral hydrate given as syrup or as dichloralphenazone (Welldorm) 650–1300 mg is suitable (see chapter 10). Barbiturates should be avoided. Other possible alternatives include nitrazepam (Mogadon) 5–10 mg and chlormethiazole (Heminevrin) 0·5–1·0 g.

Dysmnesic syndrome (Korsakoff's psychosis)

Although profound memory disturbance occurs in acute confusional states and in dementia, it is but a part, albeit an important part, of a much wider disturbance of psychological function. The term 'dysmnesic syndrome' refers to those cases in which there is a considerable impairment in the cerebral mechanism underlying the process of remembering without any clouding of consciousness (as in acute confusional state) and without any general deterioration in intellect (as in dementia). Most commonly the dysmnesic syndrome follows Wernicke's encephalopathy, itself a consequence of chronic alcoholism. When this happens the condition is synonymous with Korsakoff's psychosis; there are, however, other possible causes including encephalitis, trauma, tumours of the third ventricle and carbon monoxide poisoning. In the dysmnesic syndrome the major defect is in the retention of new information. Patients can recognise new information perfectly well, and are able to repeat it for a period of a few minutes afterwards. Yet, within a relatively short time they have no recollection of it whatsoever. The consolidation of new information into the memory store is completely blocked. Although the biochemical and physiological basis for memory is as yet ill-understood, there is greater knowledge regarding the anatomy. Bilateral lesions limited either to the mammillary bodies (as in Korsakoff's psychosis) or to the hippocampus are sufficient to produce the full clinical picture of the dysmnesic syndrome.

The inability to retain new information results in patients becoming disoriented in time and space so that they may not remember such things as the day of the month or where they are. Many patients realise their deficiencies in this regard and when pressed will invent answers to fill the gaps (confabulation). Such confabulation is, however, not an essential component of the syndrome. It has been suggested that long-term memory storage is associated with subtle alterations of chemical substances within the brain. As ribose nucleic acid (RNA) was thought to be involved, attempts have been made to provide extra RNA to patients with the dysmnesic syndrome in the hope of improving their capacity to remember. Thus far the results of such attempts have been equivocal, and any improvement noted did not appear to be permanent.

Suggestions for further reading

BERGMAN, K., 'The epidemiology of senile dementia', *British Journal of Hospital Medicine*, Vol. 1, pp. 727–32, 1969.

CORSELLIS, J. A. N., *Mental illness and the ageing brain*, Maudsley Monograph No. 9, Oxford University Press, London, 1962.

LISHMAN, W. A., 'Amnesic syndromes and their neuropathology', *Recent Developments in Psychogeriatrics*, D. W. K. Kay and A. Walk (eds), *British Journal of Psychiatry*, Special Publication No. 6, 1971.

ROTH, M., and MYERS, D. H., 'The diagnosis of dementia', *British Journal of Hospital Medicine*, Vol. 1, pp. 705–17, 1969.

WOLFF, H. G., and CURRAN, D., 'Nature of delirium and allied states', *Archives of Neurology and Psychiatry*, Vol. 33, pp. 1175–1215, 1935.

9 Personality disorders, alcoholism and drug dependence

The personality of an individual refers to that special combination of psychological traits which make him the particular person he is. It can be considered in much the same way as his physical constitution, which again is a unique amalgam of anatomical and physiological features.

While we can accurately measure such anatomical features (e.g. height), we are far less able to quantify the various personality traits. We are even uncertain about the number of traits involved. Nevertheless, personality theorists generally agree that the following are among the more important characteristics: neuroticism (anxiety-prone); obsessionality (meticulous); tendency to hysterical behaviour (self-centred, histrionic); psychopathy (antisocial); extraversion/introversion; reliability; independence.

All of us exhibit these traits to some degree; where we differ from one another is in the quantity, rather than the quality, by which they are expressed.

Personality traits can best be considered as continuous rather than discrete variables. For instance we are all somewhat prone to be anxious (i.e. neurotic); but, while some people are made anxious by the least disturbance in the environment, others hardly turn a hair, even in what to many would be a most alarming situation. The majority feel anxious in what would be generally accepted as anxiety-provoking circumstances such as examinations, job interviews and public performances. It is only when anxiety becomes extreme, or occurs under minimal stress, that treatment is indicated (see chapter 7).

Similarly, social conformity varies from one person to another: at one extreme is the self-sacrificing, saint-like person, at the other is the selfish, inconsiderate bully. It is this latter group to which the term *psychopath* or sociopath generally refers. Psychopathy is but one of the so-called personality disorders (character

148

disorders). Others include: (1) the hysterical personality (self-centred, histrionic and unreliable); (2) the dependent personality (unable to function independently, weak, easily led); (3) the obsessional personality (extremely meticulous and conscientious); (4) the explosive personality (unpredictable, given to violent outbursts); (5) the paranoid personality (suspicious, always ready to take offence); (6) the schizoid (introvert) personality (introspective, shy, sometimes aloof and emotionally cold); (7) the anxiety-prone (neurotic) personality (worries about everything). It is only when the abnormality of personality causes actual suffering to the individual concerned, or to society in general, that the term 'disorder' is justified.

Unfortunately, treatment has relatively little to offer in terms of 'cure'. Indeed, the very concept of cure is misconceived in this group of patients; we might just as well speak of 'curing' someone with an IQ of 70. All we can do is to help the patient get along with the psychological constitution (personality and intelligence) he has. Certainly by the time adulthood is reached, there is little, if any, hope of significantly influencing personality; we cannot turn the chronic worrier into a devil-may-care sort of fellow, nor can we easily transfer the callous psychopath into a model citizen. We may, however, through a psychotherapeutic approach, allow the patient to appreciate how his (or her) personality tends to produce or exacerbate certain situations, and how he or she affects other people. In addition, newer behavioural techniques offer great promise in this direction.

As far as drug-treatment is concerned, the possibilities are limited. We may afford symptomatic relief to the anxiety-prone individual, and to some degree to the chronic hypochondriacs, with anxiolytic-sedative drugs of the benzodiazepine type (see chapter 7). Other personality disorders are less amenable to drug treatment. Although claims have been made that pericyazine or propericiazine (Neulactil), a phenothiazine derivative, effectively reduces violent antisocial behaviour in those of a psychopathic personality, the claims are largely unsubstantiated by controlled experiments, and should, therefore, be accepted with caution.

Severe obsessional symptoms may be helped by administration of a tricyclic antidepressant (see chapter 6). A member of this group of drugs, clomipramine (Anafranil), has been specifically tested for its ability to alleviate obsessional disorder. Administration may be intravenous (up to 250 mg clomipramine in normal saline or 5 per cent dextrose infused over a period of one to two hours), or oral, 75 to 450 mg daily in divided doses. Although initial results from uncontrolled trials appear encouraging, enthusiasm must be tempered until results from double-blind studies are reported.

Finally, certain patterns of abnormal behaviour, including sexual deviation, alcoholism and drug dependence, are reflections of an underlying personality disorder. The place of drug treatment in the management of sexual deviation is discussed in chapter 11, while alcoholism and drug dependence are considered in the following two sections of this chapter.

Alcoholism

An alcoholic may be defined as an individual who causes problems for himself, or creates difficulties for others, by reason of excessive drinking. Although the detailed pattern of alcohol consumption may vary from patient to patient, no resolution of these problems and difficulties is likely to take place without a drastic overall reduction of alcohol intake. Alcoholism is extremely prevalent in most Western societies; in the UK the estimated total number approaches half a million. The situation in the USA is even worse; there, according to some authorities, about five million can be described as alcoholics, at an annual cost to the community of over a billion dollars.

The exact place of drug treatment in this condition has not yet been clearly established. It would appear to be of considerable benefit in the withdrawal phase, of probable benefit in some patients as a deterrent to further drinking, and of possible benefit in reducing the desire for alcohol in abstinent ex-alcoholics.

Withdrawal symptoms

When someone who has been regularly consuming large quantities of alcohol suddenly stops drinking altogether, he may well experience withdrawal symptoms, whch are a consequence of physical dependence on the drug. These can vary from mild nausea, tremulousness, headaches and general malaise to frank delirium tremens.

When mild, these symptoms usually require little more than a period of rest, together with one of the benzodiazepine drugs, either chlordiazepoxide (Librium) 10–25 mg or diazepam (Valium) 5–10 mg three times daily; an equally effective alternative is chlormethiazole (Heminevrin) 1–1·5 g two or three times daily. In contrast, the serious condition of frank delirium tremens calls for much more vigorous treatment. Clinical management includes the recognition and treatment of any concurrent medical condition, and the maintenance of an adequate fluid balance. In some cases emergency measures to counter profound hypothermia or severe hypotension may be necessary; in any case a regular watch must be maintained on temperature, pulse and blood pressure.

Treatment of the delirium itself is with large intramuscular doses of chlordiazepoxide, up to 50 mg on the first day, followed by an oral dose of up to 25 mg four times daily. Diazepam is equally effective. Paraldehyde can be given, up to 10 mg every four hours on the first day, and every six hours on the second day, followed by 20 mg at night on subsequent days. A third suitable alternative is chlormethiazole, given in an initial dose of up to 2 g.

As many patients who have reached this stage in their condition have long-standing nutritional deficiencies, it is not unreasonable to administer large doses of high-potency vitamins systemically, although it should be appreciated that there is no evidence to suggest that vitamins are in any way a specific remedy for delirium tremens.

Deterrence from further drinking

Quite by chance, two doctors who had been taking disulfiram (Antabuse) in the course of an investigation into its possible use as an antihelminthic, experienced a series of extremely unpleasant physical reactions after attending a cocktail party. They were quick to conclude that the drug they had been taking had interfered with their metabolism of alcohol thus producing a toxic reaction; disulfiram by itself had produced no such ill-effects. As a result of this observation, disulfiram was given to selected alcoholics, who although they wished to stop drinking lacked the necessary resolve to persevere. They knew that if they drank after taking disulfiram they would experience marked ill-effects, due to the presence of acetaldehyde in their circulation. The serum acetaldehyde level rises because disulfiram competes with the acetaldehyde formed from the metabolism of alcohol for the enzyme acetaldehyde dehydrogenase. The competitive inhibition of this enzyme causes the blood level of acetaldehyde to rise, producing a syndrome characterised by widespread vasodilation, (causing a violent throbbing sensation), vomiting, chest pain and dyspnoea. In addition there is a pronounced fall in blood pressure, leading to vertigo, blurred vision, and eventual collapse. The rationale behind such treatment is the hope that, in order to avoid the acetaldehyde syndrome, an alcoholic will desist from drinking once he has taken his daily disulfiram. As long as he continues to take it the potential effect will remain; however, if the patient stops taking his daily disulfiram, within a week all its effects will have worn off, and he will feel no symptoms of the acetaldehyde syndrome no matter how much he may drink. Unfortunately, this approach helps only that relatively small proportion of alcoholics whose resolve is sufficient to ensure regular administration of their disulfiram, but who without their deterrent might weaken during the course of the day. Some intrepid patients even 'drink through' their acetaldehyde reaction, potentially a highly dangerous procedure. Because of this possibility patients must be very carefully selected before being placed on a disulfiram treatment programme.

In order to familiarise patients with the risks they may run by drinking through disulfiram, it is usual to give the patients an experience of the acetaldehyde reaction before they leave hospital. Disulfiram, 1 g daily, is taken for five days; on the fifth day 18 g alcohol (equivalent to 60 ml whisky) is given. About an hour later the patient experiences the full force of the acetaldehyde syndrome. Not only is this a subjectively wretched experience, it can prove physically dangerous, so most careful nursing observation is required throughout. Should the blood pressure fall significantly the foot of the patient's bed must be raised immediately, and urgent measures taken to improve circulatory efficiency, including the intravenous administration of vasoconstrictor substances and the systemic administration of antihistamines.

Although disulfiram by itself was originally thought to be without ill-effect, experience has revealed that depression, malaise, bad-breath (due to a garlic-like flavour), impotence, gastrointestinal symptoms, and occasionally peripheral neuropathy may be produced by the drug, particularly at a dose level higher than 0·5 g per day. Because of these effects many patients are reluctant to persist in taking disulfiram for a sufficient length of time, and consequently relapse. There is also evidence that it may influence the anticoagulant activity of warfarin and interfere with prothrombin control. The usual daily dose is 100–200 mg.

As an alternative, a citrated calcium carbimide (Abstem, Temposil) which produces similar effects in combination with alcohol has the advantage of being much more rapidly metabolised and thus less likely to produce unwanted side-effects. The required dose is 50–100 mg per day.

The reduction of craving

Claims have been made that metronidazole (Flagyl) significantly reduces the craving for alcohol experienced by many alcoholics. While the earlier enthusiastic reports were not substantiated by relatively short-term controlled trials, the results from a recent twelve-month study indicated that patients taking metronidazole regularly in a dose of 600 mg daily did better than patients on placebo; 31 per cent or more in the active drug group were classified as 'improved' after twelve months compared to 3·5 per cent of those in the placebo group. It is thought that the drug acts by reducing anxiety, and by altering the taste of alcohol. The use of such an approach is somewhat limited, for patients who conscientiously persist in taking medication for such a relatively long period are hardly typical of alcoholic patients as a whole.

Therefore, while long-term drug therapy of either the deterrent type or the metronidazole type may help some alcoholics, the great majority require repeated or continuous psychological and social support; the part which drugs can play in the long-term management of this condition is at present very limited.

Finally, it should not be forgotten that some individuals are what might be considered symptomatic drinkers; that is, they drink excessively only when they become depressed as part of an affective disorder or develop symptoms of acute anxiety. In every case of alcoholism an attempt should be made to recognise any such precipitating factors; if present they should be treated promptly. Alleviation of any underlying depression (see chapter 6) or anxiety state (see chapter 7) will often reduce the patient's need to consume the alcohol which he had previously required for relief of his psychological distress.

Dependence on opiate drugs

Dependence on drugs of the opiate group, (morphine, diamorphine, methadone) is now a major social problem in many societies, particularly in the USA, where it has reached epidemic proportions (see chapter 4).

While drug treatment plays a relatively minor part in the overall management of this condition (in the UK at least), it is of considerable use when dealing with withdrawal symptoms. Furthermore the substitution of oral methadone for intravenous diamorphine (heroin) has been widely advocated as the best way of coping with the situation, although the considerable disadvantages of substituting one narcotic for another are becoming more generally recognised. A third area in which drug treatment may be of some limited use is in the maintenance of abstinence, although continued social and psychological support is likely to be of more lasting value.

The management of withdrawal

In the recently established treatment centres in Great Britain drug withdrawal is a gradual process usually undertaken under outpatient conditions. Under these circumstances there is no appearance of the classical withdrawal symptoms: lacrimation, rhinorrhoea, yawning, pilo-erection and perspiration; proceeding to extreme restlessness, violent cramp-like pains, retching and vomiting, accompanied by tachycardia and raised blood pressure. However, when the drug is stopped abruptly, then the clinical picture of withdrawal, as just described, is not only extremely distressing, but it may prove harmful also, and requires urgent treatment. Pharmacologically, the withdrawal symptoms can be terminated by administration of the drug to which the patient is addicted, but in most situations this is unlikely to be desirable, even if possible. A compound which has a similar pharmacological spectrum to heroin, such as methadone (Physeptone), can be given orally at a starting dose of 20–30 mg. This is often given with diazepam 10–20 mg. Over the next few days the dose of methadone can be reduced by 20 per cent per day, with only minimal symptoms of withdrawal.

Psychological factors play a large part in the manifestation of the withdrawal syndrome and a supportive reassuring approach can often itself greatly reduce the severity of the symptoms experienced.

An alternative regime employs a combination of diphenoxylate and atropine (Lomotil) together with chlormethiazole (Heminevrin). The diphenoxylate, which is a congener of pethidine, reduces the physical symptoms while the chlormethiazole relieves any anxiety the addict may feel regarding withdrawal. Dosage is as follows: diphenoxylate 2·5 to 5·0 mg (1–2 tablets of Lomotil) and chlormethiazole 1·0 to 2·0 g (2–4 tablets of Heminevrin) four hourly throughout the working day plus nitrazepam (Mogadon) 10 mg at night if required.

Should a heroin addict appear in a doctor's surgery (office) or hospital casualty department (receiving room) showing clear physical withdrawal symptoms, he should be given methadone up to 20 mg orally and be watched while he takes it. Arrangements can then be made for him to attend an appropriate treatment centre within the next twenty-four hours.

A situation in which withdrawal symptoms may present a serious threat to life is in babies born to opiate-dependent mothers. The first signs may appear before delivery as foetal distress. Should this occur it is imperative to ensure that the mother receives sufficient opiate to counter the withdrawal symptoms in the foetus. After delivery the infant suffering from withdrawal symptoms usually presents with irritability and tremulousness, which may be accompanied by vomiting and diarrhoea, as well as yawning, sneezing, respiratory distress, excess mucous secretion and even convulsions. Prompt treatment with chlorpromazine, 1 mg/kg body weight every four hours, is essential. This dose may be gradually reduced over the course of the next four or five weeks.

Drug substitution

As it remains a crime to prescribe heroin in many countries, including the USA, medical authorities have turned to methadone as a drug which they can prescribe, and which the addict can obtain, without committing a felony. Whereas in Great Britain licensed doctors in specified treatment centres are able to prescribe heroin (albeit with stringent safeguards), American doctors cannot do this. Therefore, in the USA the addict is faced with the choice of getting heroin illegally (which demands an enormous, unceasing financial outlay often supported by criminal activities) or methadone legally. Unfortunately, substitution of one narcotic for another hardly affects the underlying problem; it merely reduces the need for the addict to indulge in criminal acts in order to pay for the drugs he needs.

Methadone substitution consists of administering a daily oral dose of methadone 80 to 200 mg. The addict is required to attend the clinic daily to obtain this medication, which lasts him throughout the twenty-four-hour period, until he is due for his next dose. Recent studies have indicated that while withdrawal effects may be expected forty-eight hours after a methadone-free period, the effects of a new derivative, l-a-acetylmethadone last longer, and administering acetylmethadone 80 mg three times a week should prove as effective as methadone daily.

Another situation where regular methadone administration is useful occurs when an addict, maintained on intravenous heroin during the day, finds that as the effect of his evening dose does not last throughout the night he gets restless in the early hours. Here methadone linctus, up to 20 mg at night, with its greater duration of action, will usually afford a good night's sleep.

Narcotic antagonists

Substitution of an allyl group for the N-methyl group in morphine and morphine-like substances often leads to antagonism of the parent group of compounds. For instance nalorphine hydrobromide (Lethidrone) and nalorphine hydrochloride (Nalliñe) which are n-allyl morphine salts and naloxone (Narcan) which is n-allyl-diamorphine are potent morphine and heroin antagonists. When nalorphine, 1–3 mg is administered subcutaneously to someone who has recently taken a substantial dose of a narcotic drug, acute withdrawal symptoms will be experienced within fifteen minutes; these reach a peak within an hour, and persist for at least two hours. It has been suggested that the narcotic antagonists act by competing for receptor sites within the body. Cyclazocine has a similar mode of action.

These substances have been used in the supportive treatment of abstinent ex-addicts in much the same way as disulfiram is used in alcoholism. The abstinent ex-addict is advised to take daily cyclazocine 4–6 mg daily; he then knows that if he subsequently takes heroin or methadone he will experience withdrawal symptoms. Unfortunately, as with disulfiram in alcoholism, only a minority of the patients, who are insufficiently motivated to maintain abstinence without any drug, are sufficiently conscientious in their self-medication to persist for long enough.

There has recently been a suggestion that the beta-adrenergic blocking compound propranolol (see chapter 7) not only produces similar withdrawal symptoms when taken in combination with an opiate, but also markedly reduces any craving for heroin an ex-addict may have. The significance of this claim must await further confirmation before being fully accepted.

Suggestions for further reading

EDWARDS, G., 'The meaning and treatment of alcohol dependence', *Hospital Medicine*, Vol. 2, pp. 272–81, 1967.

OFFICE OF HEALTH ECONOMICS, *Drug Addiction*, London, 1967.

SCHNEIDER, K., *Psychopathic Personalities*, Cassell, London, 1958.

STEINBERG, H., *Scientific Basis of Drug Dependence*, Churchill, London, 1969.

Sleep disturbance

Nature of sleep

Although sleep is an activity which occupies about one third of our life, its nature is still poorly understood. The notion that sleep is a state analogous to suspended animation, a state of cellular inactivity, was exploded when electroencephalographic records taken during sleep showed persistent electrical activity, but of a different character to that seen in the waking state. Furthermore, experiments in which subjects have been woken at frequent intervals have suggested that some sort of mental activity can go on all through the night, but that it is almost entirely, if not completely, forgotten on waking.

The timing of sleep in the rhythm of the day's activity is learnt rather than inborn. The sleep of newborn babies tends to be regulated more by their feeding schedule than by the clock. After this early period of life, however, sleep, in common with other factors such as body temperature and diuretic activity, is governed by a twenty-four-hour rhythm. This in turn probably depends on the effects of alteration of light and darkness on hypothalamic centres which then influence hormonal activities in other parts of the body through the pituitary gland. Fast air travel across the world has emphasised the importance of our learnt diurnal sleep rhythm. Many travellers find that it takes several days to adjust their sleeping habits when they make journeys across the Atlantic or further afield.

Even if some mental activity continues during sleep, there is no doubt that a sleeping person is in a state of inertia, being unresponsive to outside events, and that a large part of the mental activity which occurs is forgotten on waking. Electroneurophysiological studies in animals have shown that the reticular formation in the brain stem is intimately concerned with the state of consciousness and responsiveness. When the reticular formation is destroyed, leaving intact the main sensory pathways to the cerebral cortex, animals are in a perpetual sleep, confirmed by the EEG, even though sensory inpulses from the periphery still reach the cortex. When, on the other hand, sensory tracts to the cortex are divided above their afferent branches to the reticular formation, the animals sleep at intervals, but may be awakened by a stimulus such as noise. They waken spontaneously and are fully active between their sleep periods. If *consciousness* implies an awareness of a recognised stimulus and the ability to respond to it, then this is not possible without a cerebral cortex, and these latter animals cannot be said to be conscious. *Wakefulness*, however, is not the same as consciousness and is possible without a cerebral cortex. It is primarily dependent on the functional integrity of the reticular system.

Electrical activity of the brain in normal sleep may be divided into two phases. The first is characterised by large-amplitude, low-frequency waves at one to three cycles per second in which sleep is profound ('slow wave sleep', 'orthodox sleep'). Brief bursts of faster activity at about twelve cycles per second are generally mixed in with these slow waves and are known as 'sleep spindles'.

The second phase, which occurs at intervals between periods of orthodox sleep, consists of low-amplitude, high-frequency, 'sawtooth' waves, accompanied by rapid conjugate movements of the eyes ('activated sleep', 'dream sleep', 'paradoxical sleep', 'rapid eye movement—REM sleep'). Respiration, heart rate and blood pressure are irregular and the penis may be erect during this phase. If subjects are wakened while their EEG record shows evidence of paradoxical sleep activity, they usually report that they were dreaming vividly. When wakened during orthodox sleep they are more likely to report 'thinking' without emphasis on imagery, action or emotion. This phase occupies in all about a quarter of the total night's sleep, recurring about five times during the night.

Electroneurophysiologists have further divided orthodox sleep into four stages. Stage 1 is the lightest phase in which subjects are most easily wakened. As sleep deepens, the EEG waves become slower and larger, reaching a maximum in Stage-4 sleep which appears the most intense and from which it is most difficult to rouse the subject. Stages 3 and 4 occur mainly in the early part of the night, and are most apparent in subjects who have been deprived of sleep. It has been suggested that orthodox sleep is associated particularly with general tissue restoration, as athletes tend to have more Stage-3 and 4 sleep on nights after strenuous physical exercise. Paradoxical sleep, on the other hand, has been related to synthetic and restorative functions in the brain, because of the increase in cerebral blood flow which accompanies it, and because of its association with the neonatal period when brain growth is rapid; it appears proportionately less in mental defect and in senility, when synthetic processes in the brain are impaired.

Hypnotism

Despite widespread misconceptions to the contrary, a subject in a so-called hypnotic trance is not asleep. Many studies have shown that the pulse and respiration rate, blood pressure, cerebral blood flow and skeletal muscle reflexes are all characteristic of the waking rather than sleeping state. These observations are confirmed by the EEG which shows a waking record.

Effects of drugs on sleep

A large number of drugs influence sleep. Central-stimulant compounds, such as caffeine, theobromine, amphetamine and its derivatives, produce varying degrees of insomnia with a reduction in total duration of night sleep, while central-depressant compounds such as barbiturate drugs induce sleep and prolong its duration. The effects of centrally acting drugs on the electrophysiological phases of sleep are more complex, however. Both central stimulant and depressant compounds reduce the proportion of time spent in paradoxical sleep. Therapeutic doses of pentobarbitone, amphetamine, phenmetrazine, methylphenidate, tranylcypromine and diethylpropion all reduce the proportion of the time spent in paradoxical sleep to between 14 and 18 per cent of total sleeping time. Alcohol, too, depresses paradoxical sleep in normal subjects. Combinations of a barbiturate with amphetamine, for example in the proprietary preparation 'Drinamyl', produce an even more marked reduction in paradoxical sleep than either constituent alone. When these centrally acting drugs are withdrawn after chronic administration there is a rebound period during which there is an increased proportion of the night spent in paradoxical sleep, particularly at the beginning of the night. Oswald has suggested that suppression of paradoxical sleep and the rapid appearance, upon withdrawal, of paradoxical sleep rebound are characteristic of drugs which lead to dependence and abuse. He has also suggested that the slow return of brain function to normal as measured by the EEG sleep pattern, which may take up to five or six weeks after withdrawal of a hypnotic drug, indicates that protein synthesis is required for the reformation of neuronal 'machinery' altered by the drug during the period of administration.

The role of neurotransmitter substances in producing various stages of sleep is still uncertain and the evidence conflicting. Non-specific reduction of brain 5HT and noradrenaline levels in animals by reserpine reduces both orthodox and paradoxical sleep. Parachlorophenylalanine, a selective inhibitor of 5HT synthesis, markedly decreases paradoxical sleep in man, while orthodox sleep remains either unchanged or is slightly increased. This is in contrast to its effects in other mammals in which orthodox sleep is decreased. Monoamine oxidase inhibitors, such as tranylcypromine, which increase tissue concentrations of 5HT and noradrenaline, lead to a progressive reduction in paradoxical sleep and increase in orthodox sleep, both in man and experimental animals. Intracerebral or intraventricular injections of 5HT or 5HTP in animals similarly lead to an increase in the time spent in orthodox sleep at the expense of paradoxical sleep. Although these studies appear to implicate 5HT in the regulation of sleep, other investigations have suggested that paradoxical sleep can be initiated or sustained by cholinergic drugs, and can be blocked or reduced by anticholinergic drugs, and stimulated by noradrenaline or its precursor dopa. Gamma-aminobutyric acid and certain short-chain fatty acids also induce sleep when injected parenterally under suitable conditions.

Prolonged hypnotic effects and hangover

An ideal hypnotic drug should not only induce sleep rapidly and predictably and maintain sleep for a reasonable length of time without influencing the ratio of orthodox to paradoxical sleep, but it should also be free from prolonged central effects. In most comparative studies of hypnotic drugs, the incidence of persistent 'hangover' effects has been assessed retrospectively and without objective tests to confirm their duration. In recent years, however, investigations have been carried out into the duration of central depression produced. Quinalbarbitone 200 mg given at bedtime was found to impair performance in a battery of psychological tests up to fifteen hours later. In other studies, nitrazepam 5 and 10 mg, and amylobarbitone sodium 100 and 200 mg were studied thirteen hours after administration to subjects who abstained from central stimulants such as caffeine. Although the subjects considered themselves alert, behavioural and psychomotor tests showed significant impairment. Further investigations showed that hypnotic doses of nitrazepam or a barbiturate impaired performance twelve hours after administration, even if subjects were allowed their usual intake of coffee or tea. These results are not surprising when it is considered that the half-lives of barbiturate hypnotic drugs and nitrazepam are between ten and twenty hours in most subjects. It is therefore important when these drugs are prescribed to warn patients of the probability of diminished efficiency on the following day, particularly in relation to driving and other skills. EEG changes due to hypnotic drugs persist very much longer than impairment of psychomotor function.

Withdrawal of hypnotic drugs

Few responsible people would dissent from the view that dependence on hypnotic drugs is undesirable and that the present increase in such dependence should be reversed. Where possible, patients dependent on these drugs should be weaned off them, but it appears that this process should be carried out gradually rather than abruptly. The sudden withdrawal of hypnotic drugs produces a 'rebound' increase in paradoxical sleep and recent investigations have suggested that some organic disease states, such as angina and myocardial ischaemia, gastric hyper-acidity and peptic ulceration, may be exacerbated during periods of increased paradoxical sleep. Caution should be exercised, therefore, in withdrawal of hypnotic drugs in patients with coronary artery disease or a history of peptic ulceration. Furthermore, abrupt withdrawal of barbiturates and occasionally of the benzodiazepines, can lead to convulsions.

Treatment of insomnia

Difficulty in sleeping is an extremely common complaint, as witnessed by the vast numbers of various sorts of sleeping tablets prescribed. It is estimated that some 600 million tablets or capsules are taken annually in the UK while the consumption in the USA is ten times as great. Of increasing importance is the frequency with which overdosage from sedative drugs occurs. With these factors in mind it should hardly be necessary to emphasise how important it is to avoid over-enthusiastic medication for what is, after all, a condition which itself carries no risk.

Before deciding on a course of treatment it is necessary to determine the causes of the sleep disturbance. Basically these are of four types:

(i) Secondary to some other condition producing discomfort, adequate treatment of which is the obvious first approach.

(ii) Environmental change in working patterns, or rapid shift from one time-zone to another as occurs in long-distance air travel. Shift workers who have to adjust to sleeping during the day one week, only to revert back to nocturnal sleeping the following week, may find it difficult to go to sleep for a night or two after changing shifts. Here, cautious and limited use of a hypnotic preparation is not unreasonable. A similar approach can be used for those travellers who may take a little while to adjust their diurnal rhythm to their new surroundings.

Another common environmental cause is having to sleep in strange surroundings, particularly in hospital, where an unfamiliar bed, the general unease felt by most when in hospital, and the noise made by other patients, all combine to prevent a good night's sleep. This is of course well recognised by medical and nursing staff. Some may consider that it is rather too well recognised in that it has become almost standard practice to prescribe night-time sedation for all patients before it is known whether or not they require it. Such practice is potentially harmful as many former patients become chronically dependent on sleeping tablets as a direct result of having first been given them while in hospital.

(iii) Certain illnesses are characterised by sleep disturbance which is an integral part of the condition. The most common such condition seen in psychiatric practice is depressive illness (endogenous depression), where early morning wakening is frequent. Patients describe how, although they can go to sleep without too much trouble, they waken in the early hours of the morning and are unable to go to sleep again. Their depression is often particularly severe at this time and the risk of suicide consequently high. It has been suggested that this change in the sleeping pattern may be related to the changes in ACTH secretion which occur in depressive illness with the morning peak coming some two to three hours earlier than normal.

Although hypnotic drugs may help to relieve the early morning wakening, treatment of the underlying depressive illness will obviously be the first step in management (see chapter 6).

(iv) By far the most common cause of sleeping difficulty is worry or emotional strain: mothers worried about their children, husbands concerned over their job, adolescents crossed in love. All can lie awake, tossing and turning, brooding over their problems.

Eventually they nearly always get off to sleep, but do not feel refreshed when they waken to face their problems again. In many such cases frank discussion of their fears and worries may itself relieve the tension sufficiently to render any pharmacological intervention unnecessary.

Before any prescription for sedative drugs is given to a patient, he should be warned against the possible synergistic effects of alcohol, and should be cautioned against drinking shortly before, or after, taking his night sedation.

Finally, doctors should be sparing in the quantity of tablets or capsules prescribed at one time, thus minimising the risk of overdosage; similarly, they should be cautious in the frequency with which they prescribe hypnotic drugs to any one patient, thus minimising the risk of dependence.

Choice of therapy

There are two main categories of hypnotic drugs: barbiturates and non-barbiturates (see Table 7).

1 *Barbiturates* Although barbiturate compounds have several potential disadvantages they have the one great advantage of being well-tested by time. Furthermore, the non-barbiturate hypnotics share most of the disadvantages of the barbiturates with the added factor that far less is known about their metabolism, and perhaps more importantly, about their possible ill-effects. The thalidomide tragedy is a stark reminder of this.

Provided that the cautions mentioned above are observed, the barbiturates probably remain among the most useful preparations for the treatment of insomnia in otherwise healthy adults. In the elderly, however, they can cause confusion, and here a non-barbiturate alternative is preferable. Furthermore patients in whom the risk of over-dosage is high, that is, patients with marked depressive features or patients with a previous history of attempted suicide, may also be less at risk with a non-barbiturate alternative. Their other side-effects are discussed in Chapter 7.

Among the barbiturates there is very little to choose from among those listed in Table 7. They all have more or less the same duration of action and all require to be taken in approximately the same dosage. In most cases 100 mg taken one hour before retiring will be sufficient, although in some patients, particularly where anxiety is intense, 200 mg may be required. There is no advantage to be gained from a mixture of barbiturates, or from a mixture of other drugs with a barbiturate. Where reliable trials have been conducted into the efficacy of such mixtures, it has invariably been found that it is the barbiturate content which counts.

2   *Non-barbiturates*   Of the non-barbiturate hypnotic compounds listed in the table, three groups deserve special mention:

(i) *Chloral hydrate*   This is a relatively weak hypnotic which, when absorbed, is metabolised to trichlorethanol. Its main disadvantage is its unpleasant taste and it also has an unfortunate tendency to produce gastric irritation. It should therefore be taken well-diluted with milk or olive oil. The preparation, dichloralphenazone (Welldorm), which is in tablet form, may be a more acceptable way of administering the same compound, being particularly useful in the elderly.

(ii) *Methaqualone*   Taken by itself this too is only moderately effective. However it is greatly potentiated by the addition of the antihistamine diphenhydramine (Benadryl), as in the preparation 'Mandrax', so much so that the rapidity of onset may prove embarrassing if the patient is not forewarned. This quick action makes it particularly favoured by drug-abusers, and as a result widespread dependency problems have arisen in the United Kingdom. In addition, overdosage, which is often accompanied by convulsions, can prove very difficult to treat. For these reasons the methaqualone and diphenhydramine mixture should be used with great caution, if at all.

(iii) *Benzodiazepine derivatives*   Certain members of the anxiolytic sedative drugs, the benzodiazepines, for example, chlordiazepoxide (Librium) have been found to have marked hypnotic

165

properties. Nitrazepam (Mogadon) and flurazepam (Dalmane) are both marketed for their sedative properties. They have the same mode of action and can be considered together. While they produce hypnotic effects similar to the barbiturates and lead to just as prolonged impairment of the psychomotor skills, they do have the great advantage of safety. Over-dosage is very rarely fatal, a point of particular relevance when treating potential suicides. Furthermore liver enzyme induction does not occur.

Continuous sedation

Some psychiatrists find that continuous sedation, or 'sleep treatment', may be of value in severe, prolonged anxiety states, although the efficacy of this approach has never been rigorously tested. The aim is to keep the patient asleep for the greater part of the day over a period of several days. Large doses of barbiturates (200–300 mg three or four times a day) are required, and skilled nursing care is needed to prevent respiratory complications or pressure sores. Physical dependence to barbiturates can occur if the treatment goes on long enough and withdrawal fits can provide an added complication.

Narcolepsy

In this condition, the pathogenesis of which remains obscure, patients are frequently overtaken by irresistible attacks of sleep from which they can be readily wakened. Attacks, which may occur several times in one day are characteristically brought on in susceptible individuals by emotional arousal. Narcolepsy is probably the only condition in adults for which administration of amphetamine is justified. It can be given either as the racemic mixture amphetamine sulphate (Benzedrine) or as the dextrorotatory-isomer, dexamphetamine sulphate (Dexedrine), both in a dosage of 5–10 mg three or four times a day. Milder degrees of narcolepsy may respond to caffeine, either given as tablets (100–300 mg), or taken in coffee.

Table 7 *Hypnotics*

Approved name	*Proprietary name*	*Recommended dose*	*Remarks*
barbiturates			
amylobarbitone sodium (UK) amobarbital (USA)	Sodium Amytal	100–200 mg	Well tried, effective hypnotics. Can produce confusion in the elderly and drug dependence in the susceptible. Over-dosages frequently fatal. Not too much to choose between them. All relatively cheap
butobarbitone (UK) butobarbital (USA)	Soneryl	100–200 mg	
heptabarbitone (UK) heptabarbital (USA)	Medomin	200 mg	
pentobarbitone (UK) pentobarbital (USA)	Nembutal	50–100 mg	
quinalbarbitone (UK) secobarbital (USA)	Seconal	50–100 mg	
quinalbarbitone and amylobarbitone	Tuinal	100–200 mg	No advantage over its constituents prescribed singly
non-barbiturates			
carbromal (and pento-barbitone 100 mg)	Carbrital	250 mg	Efficacy almost entirely attributable to barbiturate content
chloral hydrate trichlorethyl phosphate	Somnos Triclofos	1–2 g well-diluted	Safe, particulary useful in the elderly. Unpleasant taste with tendency to produce gastric irritation
dichloral-phenazone	Welldorm	650–1300 mg	Relatively weak hypnotic, useful in elderly

Table 7—*Contd.*

Approved name	Proprietary name	Recommended dose	Remarks
ethchlorvynol	Arvynol Serenesil Placidyl	250–500 mg	Equally effective as barbiturates and glutethamide. Seems safe and relatively cheap
ethinamate	Valmid	500 mg	Short-acting. Useful for initiating sleep. Little hangover effects
glutethimide	Doriden	250–500 mg	Although classified as non-barbiturate efficacy and side-effects similar. May be excreted more rapidly with less prolonged effects
meprobamate	Equanil, Miltown	400–800 mg	Good in the elderly
methaqualone (and diphenhydramine 25 mg)	Quaalude Mandrax	150–300 mg 250 mg	Moderately effective Rapid onset of action. Considerable tendency to produce dependence. Over-dosage difficult to treat
methyprylone	Noludar Noctan Dimerin	200–300 mg	Actions and toxic effects similar to chloral hydrate
nitrazepam	Mogadon	5–10 mg	⎫ Effective and relatively
flurazepam	Dalmane	15–30 mg	⎬ safe although likely to ⎭ produce hangover effects

Suggestions for further reading

CLIFT, A. D., 'Factors leading to dependence on hypnotic drugs', *British Medical Journal*, Vol. 3, pp. 614–17, 1972.

OSWALD, I., 'Drugs and sleep', *Pharmacological Reviews*, Vol. 20, pp. 273–303, 1968.

'Sleeping pills: the day after' (anon.), *Drug and Therapeutics Bulletin*, Vol. 9, pp. 9–10, 1971.

Sexual problems

Physiology of sexual behaviour

The study of human sexual function can best be considered under two headings: drive and performance.

Sexual drive

The drive towards sexual activity has both strength and direction, and is largely under the control of the central nervous system. While the strength of sexual drive can be markedly influenced by physiological and pharmacological factors, the direction it takes in man is almost entirely determined by psychological and social influences.

In contrast, the direction of sexual behaviour of lower mammals is markedly influenced by pituitary function. For instance, in the guinea pig an injection of testosterone into the developing foetus will lead to a male type of behaviour pattern in later life, whatever the gonadal sex. In rats similar effects can be obtained with testosterone injection up to fifteen days post-natally. On the other hand oestrogens have no such effects. It is therefore considered that it is the absence of androgens in the females of lower mammalian species, rather than the presence of oestrogens, which directs psychological development into characteristic female behavioural patterns. In humans, however, social factors play a much more dominant part in determining genital role. For instance, female infants born with a hyperactive adrenal gland, and a consequently high androgen level (the adrenogenital syndrome), may be confused with a male at birth, particularly because the over-developed clitoris may be mistaken for a penis. If adequate steroid therapy is instituted to reduce pituitary ACTH secretion, the adrenal androgen levels fall and normal feminisation takes place, although there may be a persistent tomboyish tendency. There seems to be little indecisiveness in subsequent gender identification and no tendency towards homosexuality in spite of the high pre-natal androgen levels, which in lower animals would have had a lasting effect. Similarly, males with pronounced hypospadias, leading to a mis-classification of gender, can develop either in the male or the female role, after plastic repair. The important thing is for the parents to be consistent in their attitude.

At puberty, development of secondary sex characteristics is dependent on gonadal activity which in turn is influenced by the pituitary. Castrated males (eunuchs) fail to develop sexually and have limited sexual interest. Replacement therapy with androgens leads to normal sexualisation and an increase in the strength of sexual drive. Stopping such medication results in a diminished ejaculatory volume, fewer erections and less sexual desire. In contrast the sexuality of females with hypogonadism is little impaired and not at all influenced by oestrogen replacement, although certain women with reduced libido may be helped by androgens (see below). Thus in both sexes it is the androgens which influence the strength of the sexual drive, but not the direction this drive will take.

Primate females undergo a regular monthly cyclic change in their output of oestrogens and progesterone, corresponding with the menstrual cycle. These fluctuations in hormone levels may in some cases be accompanied by changes in sexual responsiveness. Certainly in rhesus monkeys the sexual activity reaches its maximum at mid-cycle when ovulation occurs. This has obvious biological advantages: with the gradual rise in oestrogen and progesterone concentration which takes place in the second, or luteal, phase of the menstrual cycle, sexual activity falls. This not only directly affects the female's responsiveness, but also impairs the attractiveness of the female for the male monkey, as measured by the number of mounting attempts. Similarly, the administration of oral contraceptive preparations containing 1 mg ethynodiol diacetate and 0·05 mg mestranol to female monkeys leads to a gradual reduction in the number of ejaculations by the male. These findings suggest that at least two mechanisms underlie sexual responsiveness in monkeys. First, there is an oestrogen-dependent vaginal change which stimulates the male, probably through his sense of smell. Second, there is an oestrogen action on the central nervous system of the female, which increases her responsiveness. This view has been substantiated by ingenious conditioning experiments where it was found that oophorectomised females were not a reward for male monkeys until they had been given oestrogens.

Many human females also notice a similar waxing and waning of sexual desire during the menstrual cycle, although here the picture is more complex. For instance, oophorectomy appears to have but little effect in human sexual activity in contrast to monkeys. Nevertheless, hypophysectomy does lead to a profound fall in the level of sexual desire and satisfaction, probably due to the secondary reduction in the level of adrenal androgens. Thus, in humans, sexual behaviour takes place in response to both internal (physiological) and external (psychological and social) factors, the actual behaviour pattern being largely determined by genetic predisposition and previous experience.

Human sexual performance

Until Masters' and Johnson's recent comprehensive observations of human sexual performance under laboratory conditions, knowledge of the detailed physiological changes which take place during sexual intercourse was poorly understood. According to Masters and Johnson, the human sexual response in both sexes occurs in four more or less distinct phases: the excitement phase, the plateau phase, orgasm and, finally, resolution.

These will now be discussed for each sex separately.

Sexual performance of the male

1 *Excitement phase* This phase is characterised by penile erection. The penis consists of three cylindrical bodies of erectile tissue, which receive their blood supply from the internal pudendal arteries. When these arteries and their arterioles dilate, under the control of parasympathetic splanchnic nerves, blood fills trabeculated cavernous spaces within the erectile tissue and erection occurs. On contraction of the arterioles, under the control of the sympathetic nerves accompanying the arteries, the penis becomes flaccid.

Excess sympathetic activity, as occurs in anxiety states, will prevent penile erection and thereby hinder satisfactory sexual intercourse. Similarly malfunction or malformation of the parasympathetic nerve supply may also be a rare cause of failure of erection. Once a man has failed to obtain or maintain a satisfactory erection, the next time he attempts intercourse he is likely to be worried that he will fail. The very fact of his worrying tends to further increase sympathetic activity and prevent satisfactory penile erection. A vicious circle develops leading to the clinical condition of impotence.

2 *Plateau phase* After the erection of the penis there is an increase in tumescence.

3 *Orgasm phase* Just before orgasm a slight mucoid emission occurs which can contain motile spermatozoa. This may be a result of secretion from Cowper's glands. Almost immediately the vasa efferentia, the epididymis, the vasa deferentia, the seminal vesicles and the prostate all contract and together with the perineal muscles propel the seminal fluid rapidly through the penile urethra to the external meatus.

4 *Resolution phase* This refers to the period following orgasm before the individual is ready to commence intercourse again. The duration of this period can vary considerably.

Sexual performance of the female

1 *Excitement phase* The first physiological manifestation of sexual arousal in women is the moistening of the vaginal walls from a transudation of fluid from the plexus of veins surrounding the vagina. It is not a true secretion, as there are no glandular elements within the vaginal wall.

Shortly afterwards there is vasocongestion of the breasts and nipple erection, engorgement of the labia majora and labia minora, and some distention of the clitoris.

2 *Plateau phase* This phase is marked by a localised vasocongestion of the outer third of the vagina which later contracts strongly during orgasm.

3 *Orgasm phase* Masters and Johnson describe this phase as 'a brief episode of physical relief from the myotonic and vasocongestive increment developed in response to sexual stimuli'.

4 *Resolution phase* This tends to be of much shorter duration than in the male. In both males and females the cycle of sexual response described is possibly developed from 'a drive of biologic-behavioural origin deeply integrated into the condition of human existence'. There is, however, marked variation in the intensity and duration of the sexual response, which is to a large degree affected by social and psychological influences. Sexual fears in the female tend to be concerned either with the attainment of satisfactory orgasm or the sexual drive in general, whereas in the male sexual fears have related almost entirely to the attainment and mainte-nance of a penile erection. Not surprisingly perhaps, pharmaco-logical remedies have long been sought for these problems.

Drugs affecting sexual behaviour

Sexual desire and performance may, as we have seen, be affected by psychological factors like anxiety, by the level of circulating androgens, by the activities of the autonomic nervous system and by local stimulation of the genital tract. Drugs influencing these functions may thus have an effect on sexual behaviour.

Although from time immemorial men have sought love philtres to arouse the passion of women and to increase their own sexual powers, it is only in recent times that attempts have been de-liberately made to reduce sexual drive. Furthermore, certain centrally acting drugs used in psychiatry have the disturbing property of adversely affecting sexual performance. Also with the advent of oral contraceptives many women have noted a profound effect of these compounds on their sexuality. Each of these topics will be considered in turn.

Drugs to increase sexual drive and performance (aphrodisiacs)

Centrally acting psychotropic drugs

1 *Anxiolytic sedatives* Anxiolytic sedatives and alcohol, by reducing subjective anxiety, may lower the level of sympathetic discharge sufficiently to allow penile erection to occur in cases of impotence. The dosage is critical, however, for too high a blood level may itself inhibit the parasympathetic mechanism controlling the blood supply to the penile erectile tissue. Shakespeare's

summary of this pharmacological action of alcohol can hardly be bettered:

> Lechery, sir, it provokes, and unprovokes: it provokes the
> desire, but takes away the performance: therefore much
> drink may be said to be an equivocator with lechery: it makes
> him and it mars him; it sets him on, and it takes him off; it
> persuades him and disheartens him; makes him stand to, and
> not to stand to; in conclusion, equivocates him in a sleep, and,
> giving him the lie, leaves him.
>
> *(Macbeth, Act II, Scene 3)*

Frigidity in women is often due to an irrational anxiety about sexual intercourse. Allaying such anxiety with anxiolytic sedatives would seem to be a sensible approach to the problem. In other cases, frigidity is a reflection of social inhibitions which are frequently, it has been said, 'soluble in alcohol'.

A more specific approach to the problems of impotence and frigidity, using the techniques of behaviour therapy, has recently been devised (see chapter 7).

2 *Opiates and psychodysleptics* In the East it is still widely held that opium increases the pleasures of sexual activity, and because of its sedative action, reduces the likelihood of premature ejaculation. While this may be true for the occasional user, it is quite clear that morphine and heroin addicts are almost completely lacking in sexual drive.

LSD has been alleged to have aphrodisiac properties but this is almost certainly illusory. Rather than producing a heightening of true sexual desires, it produces what Havelock Ellis aptly called 'an orgy of vision'.

Cannabis is also endowed with aphrodisiac properties by some and is frequently taken in Egypt to improve a waning sexuality. When taken regularly, however, it has the opposite effect: 'A Romeo who took hashish would quickly have forgotten Juliet' (*Gautier*).

3 *Psychostimulants* Amphetamines, by combating fatigue and heightening desire, can occasionally prolong sexual activity. In most cases, however, they reduce potency by their sympathomimetic action.

Androgens

We have already seen how the strength of sexual drive in both sexes is determined, at least partly, by the level of circulating androgens. Androgens do not however affect reduced potency unless the impotence is a reflection of impaired testicular function. They do not influence homosexual tendencies.

Androgens have been reported as helping certain cases of frigidity in women.

Drugs acting on the autonomic system

As impotence is usually due to increased sympathetic activity, direct sympathetic inhibition might improve potency. Yohimbine, an alkaloid derived from the bark of a West African tree is an adrenergic alpha-receptor blocking agent. This might be the basis of its postulated aphrodisiac qualities, although as yet there is no direct evidence of its efficacy. Propranolol, a beta-receptor blocking agent, has been tried also in psychogenic impotence, but without success. In animals, p-chlorophenylalanine, which reduces brain levels of 5HT, appears to increase total sexual activity. As yet the effects on human sexuality remain to be investigated.

Finally, thioridazine, a phenothiazine compound (see chapter 5) possesses marked anti-adrenergic properties and has been used for premature ejaculation.

Local irritants

Cantharidin is a non-volatile anhydride present in a particular species of beetle (*Cantharis vesicatoria*), popularly called 'Spanish fly'. When ingested it irritates the gastrointestinal tract and during its excretion in the urine causes irritation of the urinary tract. It is this irritative action on the lower urinary tract which is supposed to heighten sexual desire. Whether or not it is effective, cantharidin is extremely dangerous, and fatalities have been reported.

Drugs which reduce sexual drive and performance

Oestrogens

Oestrogens can effectively reduce sexual drive in men, but this may be accompanied by irreversible gynaecomastia. Their effects in women are less predictable (see below).

Anti-androgens

Recently synthetic anti-androgen compounds have been synthesised, which are non-feminising. Cyproterone has this property and is said to be useful in suppressing sexual desire. Provera is a synthetic progestogen which antagonises testosterone. It too has been claimed to reduce libido.

Psychotropic drugs

Anxiolytic sedatives and alcohol which can, if taken in too high a dosage, lead to a reduced sexual performance, have already been discussed (see chapter 7).

Phenothiazine derivatives rarely reduce potency in men, but may well affect sexual function in women. Oligomenorrhoea, impaired ovulation and failure of uterine implantation of the fertilised ovum have all been reported. As these compounds possibly act on hypothalamic centres (see chapter 5), it is not surprising that they influence pituitary function which itself is under hypothalamic control.

Antidepressants, both the dibenzazepines as well as the mono-amine oxidase inhibitors, frequently lead to partial impotence in men.

Drugs acting on the autonomic system

Adrenergic neurone-blocking drugs, particularly guanethidine (Ismelin) and bethanidine (Esbatal), may produce impotence, but more commonly failure of ejaculation.

Psychological effects of oral contraceptives

Between a quarter and a third of all women not on oral contraceptives notice that they tend to become somewhat depressed in the two or three days preceding their menstrual period. This depression is frequently accompanied by irritability and headache and occurs at the time of the month when the levels of circulating oestrogens and progesterone reach their peak. It is known that prolonged administration of progestogens frequently leads to depressive symptoms and marked reduction in sexual drive. There have been a number of studies of the psychological effects accompanying regular monthly administration of oral contraceptive preparations containing a mixture of an oestrogenic compound with a progestogen. While some women notice a definite improvement in their mood with oral contraceptives, others complain of a pronounced worsening of premenstrual depression and loss of libido. These inconsistencies do not appear to be related to the exact nature of the oestrogens or progestogens used, or, within limits, to their relative concentrations, although some women seem to do better on one preparation than another.

Drug treatment of sexual problems

Impotence and frigidity

In the great majority of cases these symptoms are entirely psychogenic and may be improved by anxiolytic sedatives which should be taken some one or two hours before retiring. The appropriate dosage may take some time to determine, as too little will be ineffective while too much will cause sedation. Either a barbiturate such as sodium amylobarbitone 50–100 mg or a benzodiazepine derivative like diazepam 2–5 mg may be used. Often an alcoholic 'nightcap' is as effective.

If this relatively non-specific approach fails, specific desensitisation with methohexitone or propanidid should be tried (see chapter 7).

In those very rare cases which are unequivocally due to pathologically low levels of circulating androgens, testosterone propionate 5–10 mg injected once or twice a week or a testosterone implant containing 100–500 mg may be useful.

Finally, in cases where the adrenergic neurone-blocking drug bethanidine is being taken, omission of the evening dose may lead to satisfactory sexual function.

Sexual deviations

Sexual deviation is more common among men than among women, and men are more likely to commit grave antisocial acts in order to gratify their sexual desires. While no pharmacological agent can by itself alter the direction of sexual desire, oestrogens will reduce its strength. Either stilboestrol 5–10 mg daily or ethinyl oestradiol 0·02–0·05 mg daily can be used. Common side-effects include nausea and gynaecomastia. Such an approach should only be considered when the sexual deviation is causing considerable distress to the individual concerned or there is a real danger of antisocial acts being committed. It is obvious that the whole-hearted cooperation of the patient is necessary.

The anti-androgen compounds, cyproterone and provera, already referred to, offer a promising alternative to oestrogens for this purpose. The butyrophenone compound benperidol has also been reported to be effective.

An altogether different approach to sexual deviation involves the attempt to desensitise the patient to any possible anxieties he may have regarding normal heterosexual intercourse. This is based on the belief that many sexual perversions arise because of difficulties, either real or imagined, with heterosexual intercourse; relieving these difficulties should remove the need for deviant behaviour. Considerable success for this approach has been claimed in the treatment of homosexuality, particularly when combined with other behavioural techniques like aversion therapy.

Suggestions for further reading

MASTERS, W. H., and JOHNSON, V. E., *Human Sexual Response*, Churchill, London, 1966.

MICHAEL, R. P., *Endocrinology and Human Behaviour*, Oxford University Press, London, 1968

PERRY, J. S., 'Effects of pharmacologically active substances on sexual function', *Journal of Reproduction and Fertility*, Supplement No. 4, 1968.

Disorders of appetite and body weight   12

Physiology of appetite and weight regulation

The sensation of hunger, one of the major factors controlling calorie intake, plays a crucial role in the regulation of calorie balance and body weight. A constant body weight implies that calorie intake (as food) exactly balances calorie expenditure (through exercise and metabolism). The fact that body weight does remain more or less constant in most people reflects the accuracy with which calorie intake, and presumably hunger, is related to need. Only a slight variation in this relationship will, in the course of time, lead to a considerable weight change. For example, if a man weighing 70 kg, expending 3,000 K cal. per day, were regularly to consume 1 per cent more calories than he required (and this would be equivalent to a mere extra half-slice of bread and butter a day), he would more than double his weight during his working life, becoming grossly obese by the time he reached sixty-five; indeed his adiposity would greatly reduce his chances of living that long.

Hypothalamus

The key to this regulating system lies in the hypothalamus. The ventro-medial hypothalamus contains the satiety centre, and the lateral parts contain the feeding centres. After lesions are made in the medial satiety centre, experimental animals eat almost non-stop, often reaching an enormous size; they behave during this dynamic phase of weight gain as if food fails to satisfy them. Conversely if this same area is stimulated electrically then the animal will stop eating, even though it may have been deprived of food for several hours. The lateral feeding centres act reciprocally to the satiety centre: when they are destroyed, or even when the dopaminergic neurones within them are selectively killed with

179

6-hydroxdopamine all feeding behaviour stops, whereas stimulation of the feeding centres can initiate feeding in seemingly sated animals. The activity of the two centres is closely co-ordinated; from electrophysiological evidence it is likely that the spontaneous activity of the lateral feeding centres is modified by the medial satiety centre, the latter acting as a brake on the feeding centres.

There would appear to be two types of body weight regulation associated with the hypothalamus: the first is short-term and involves the calories consumed during a given meal or on a single day, while the second is long-term, determining the level of body weight over periods of weeks and months rather than days.

The short-term regulating system is concerned with the onset of feeding behaviour and its duration, together with how much is eaten on any one occasion. It is not yet known with any certainty what physiological cues affect the system, that is, what signals the hypothalamus receives to activate the feeding centre or to inhibit the satiety centre (or, in more psychological terms, what somatic events underlie the subjective sensations of hunger and satiety). Nevertheless, certain theories have been proposed. These include the *glucostatic theory*, in which blood sugar levels are the important regulators, and the *thermostatic theory*, in which ambient temperature plays a crucial role. In addition the motor activity of the stomach appears to play some part in this regulatory system.

Glucostatic theory

This theory suggests that the level of hunger experienced depends not so much on the absolute level of blood sugar, but on the concentration gradient of glucose between the arterial blood and the venous blood. A large a/v gradient reflects active glucose utilisation and storage, this implies that sufficient glucose is available; under these conditions there would be no need for further nutriment and hunger would not be felt. A narrowing of the gradient indicates a relative insufficiency of glucose, which would lead to the sensation of hunger.

While this mechanism may play some part in hunger regulation, experimental evidence suggests that it is insufficient as a complete explanation.

Thermostatic theory

In colder climates a considerable proportion of the total energy expenditure is directed towards maintaining a stable body temperature. Furthermore, people tend to eat more when it is cold than when it is warm. On the basis of these observations it has been postulated that essentially we eat to keep warm, and our eating behaviour is largely determined by our skin temperature. While it is very probable that skin temperature does play a part in the regulation of food intake, it too is unlikely to provide the complete explanation of hunger.

Gastric activity

Many, if not most, individuals have experienced abdominal sensations, often somewhat unpleasant, when they feel hungry. Such sensations are a reflection of periodic gastric contractions which occur episodically in the fasting state. While such contractions are a frequent accompaniment of subjective hunger they are by no means essential for the regulation of calorie balance, as both animals and patients who have undergone a complete gastrectomy are able to regulate their calorie balance successfully. The stomach is perhaps of greater importance in the appreciation of satiety. When we speak of feeling 'full-up' we are usually referring to a largely gastric sensation.

Psychological and social factors

In most societies the pattern of eating and the content of meals is determined more by psychological and social factors than by physiological cues. It is particularly important to bear this in mind when one is trying to alter eating habits; no matter how impressive the scientific arguments put forward to emphasise to the patient the need to change his diet, the attempt will prove futile if the patient is not suitably motivated, or if the advice given runs counter to his social expectations.

The long-term regulation of body weight is even less well understood. If this is controlled by the hypothalamus, as it seems to be, the hypothalamus must be able to detect changes in total adipose tissue, possibly through levels of circulating non-esterified fatty acids (NEFA), or perhaps through some, as yet undetected, metabolite which reflects the amount of adipose tissue in the body. It may even be that the hypothalamus can monitor the volume of adipose tissue directly.

Although hunger is one of the most fundamental motivating factors in human behaviour, our understanding of its physiological basis is, as we have seen, still very fragmentary. However, as with many other physiological functions, pharmacological inquiries have already helped to elucidate the situation, and should assist even more in the future.

Pharmacology of drugs affecting appetite

Drugs affecting appetite and food intake fall sharply into two groups: (1) those which reduce hunger—appetite suppressants or *anorectics* (2) those which increase hunger.

Appetite suppressant drugs These are of three main types: (i) drugs acting centrally on the hypothalamic centres (ii) drugs influencing carbohydrate metabolism (iii) bulk agents acting directly on the stomach.

(i) *Centrally acting compounds* Most preparations in this group are amines and include amphetamine (Benzedrine) and its dextro-rotatory isomer dexamphetamine (Dexedrine), together with phenmetrazine (Preludin), diethylpropion (Tenuate, Apisate), phentermine (Duromine), chlorphentermine (Lucofen, Presate) and fenfluramine (Ponderax, Ponderal); mazindol (Teronac), by contrast, is an indole derivative.

All these compounds when given to animals markedly reduce calorie intake, which in turn leads to weight loss. It is likely that they act on the hypothalamic feeding centres, possibly by stimulating amine receptors directly, or by releasing catecholamines from nerve endings. They do not appear to influence the a/v glucose gradient or fasting gastric motility. In human subjects there is good evidence to indicate that amphetamine, dexamphetamine, phenmetrazine, diethylpropion and fenfluramine can significantly reduce both subjective hunger, as measured by a linear analogue scale and food intake, under suitably controlled conditions; that is, they do have a true appetite suppressant action which reaches its peak some two hours after oral administration. All but fenfluramine have a distinctly stimulating action on the CNS; clinically the patients may notice an increased alertness or a reduction of fatigue, while experimentally they have been shown to increase CFF.

Fenfluramine differs somewhat from the other compounds in this group in that it has no stimulating action whatsoever on the CNS, although its anorectic action is equivalent to the others. This suggests that the appetite suppressant activity of this group of compounds is not merely secondary to central stimulation as had been proposed at one time, but is a primary action in its own right. Fenfluramine, and possibly the other drugs in this group, may have a peripheral as well as a central action. It appears to lead to an increased utilisation of glucose, which by increasing the a/v glucose gradient, might, according to the glucostatic theory, promote a reduction in the sensation of hunger.

(ii) *Drugs affecting carbohydrate metabolism*

(a) *Glucagon*   This is a hormone produced by the α cells of the pancreas which elevates blood-sugar levels and increases the a/v glucose gradient.

While glucagon does lead to a reduction in both subjective hunger and food intake in healthy subjects, as would be predicted by the glucostatic theory, the maximum effect is not observed until some two hours following intramuscular injection, occurring later than the blood-sugar effect. It may be that glucagon influences some other factor, such as gastric motility, which in turn affects the hypothalamus. Measures of gastric motility have shown that glucagon does indeed reduce motility, but again the maximum reduction in motility occurs rather earlier than the maximum hunger reduction.

(b) *Biguanides*   Two compounds in this group, metformin (Glucophage) and phenformin (Dibotin), which have a hypo-glycaemic action, are widely used in the treatment of diabetes mellitus, particularly the maturity-onset type commonly associated with obesity. It was noticed that obese diabetic patients appeared to lose weight much more easily while they were taking metformin or phenformin than on diet alone.

The mechanism by which these compounds affect body weight is obscure. In diabetics they increase the peripheral utilisation of glucose by improving the insulin clearance in muscle as compared to adipose tissue. Yet in non-diabetic obese subjects, where there is also a reduced peripheral glucose uptake, the biguanides do not improve peripheral glucose uptake, but probably act by reducing gluconeogenesis. It is debatable whether the biguanide compounds have a true anorectic action, as distinct from producing nausea.

(iii) *Bulk agents* As methylcellulose was observed to swell in the presence of water it was hoped that if it were swallowed it would similarly swell inside the stomach and thereby produce a feeling of satiety. No direct evidence of any such effect has been produced. In a series of carefully controlled observations, doses of methylcellulose of up to 3 g (9 tablets) led to no detectable reduction of either measured food intake or subjective hunger ratings. Equally, controlled clinical trials of these substances in obese subjects have failed to reveal any significant weight reduction attributable to them.

Appetite stimulating drugs

1 *Insulin* Both exogenous insulin administration and endogenous hypersecretion, as occurs in spontaneous hypoglycaemia, are accompanied by a marked increase in subjective hunger. From experimental studies it is clear that this hunger does not appear until the blood sugar has reached its lowest point and is beginning to rise, that is, some thirty minutes after administration. It may be of significance that the onset of hunger occurs at approximately the same time as the appearance of pronounced fasting gastric motility. However, it is likely that both the subjective awareness of hunger and the occurrence of gastric motility are themselves secondary to hypothalamic activity.

2 *Phenothiazines* Chlorpromazine (Largactil) and its derivatives, which are widely used in the treatment of schizophrenia (see chapter 5), frequently lead to considerable weight gain; in some series virtually all patients on continuous phenothiazine medication were noted to have gained weight, with some becoming distinctly obese. Those who develop marked adiposity report that the medication seems to make them feel voraciously hungry.

As careful studies have failed to reveal any metabolic cause for the increase in weight observed, it is likely that these compounds directly affect the hunger-regulating mechanism in the hypothalamus. Recent experimental evidence supports this view; direct injection of chlorpromazine into the hypothalamic feeding centre promoted increased food intake in animals.

3 *Cyproheptadine (Periactin)* This compound, which has anti-histaminic properties and which also antagonises the activity of 5-hydroxytryptamine, was introduced clinically as an anti-histamine. Patients receiving it were noted to gain weight and laboratory animals were shown to consume more calories when cyproheptadine was given. In addition, significant weight gain was observed in both children and adults following cyproheptadine administration, as compared to that occurring after placebo. The assumption was made that the observed increase in weight reflected an underlying rise in hunger, and a consequent increase in food intake. Evidence has recently been obtained which substantiates this view; a group of young adults were shown to feel significantly more hungry when taking cyproheptadine than when taking placebo. This effect could be related to the compound's anti-5HT activity, particularly as 5HT occurs in the hypothalamus in high concentration.

Drug treatment of appetite disorders

The two clinical conditions in which disturbances of body weight and appetite are of primary importance are obesity and psychogenic malnutrition (anorexia nervosa). In obesity there is an excess of adipose tissue, arising from more calories being consumed than are expended, while psychogenic malnutrition develops if more calories are expended than are consumed. The rational treatment of each situation is to reverse the calorie imbalance which has occurred. In both situations it is the appropriate dietary regime which is of fundamental importance; the place of drugs is secondary, they should only be used as adjuncts to dietary treatment, never as a substitute for it.

Obesity

For most clinical purposes body weight will suffice as an index of the degree of adiposity present; an individual can be considered as clinically obese if he exceeds his ideal body weight by 20 per cent. When this level of overweight is reached it is time for treatment to be instituted. Treatment should be based on appropriate dietary advice, together with an admonition to take frequent, but moderate, exercise. In most cases patients will require close supervision and support which is best provided by their family doctor seeing them initially at weekly or fortnightly intervals. Such supportive care is particularly important in those patients whose obesity is a consequence of psychological disturbance. Although such patients form a minority of the overweight subjects in the population they are usually the ones who find it the most difficult to keep to a diet. Their eating pattern is not only determined by physiological requirements; psychological needs play a great part. They find that food, particularly sweet food, helps to reduce their anxiety or depression and therefore suffer greater temptations to break their diet than the majority of obese patients who have no such underlying psychological disturbance.

Appetite suppressant drugs can in some cases provide a useful addition to combined dietary and supportive treatment, but should not be used as the sole treatment.

1 *Amphetamine* (*Benzedrine*) *and dexamphetamine* (*Dexedrine*)
Amphetamine was originally introduced as a treatment for obesity following the observation in the 1930s that a proportion of patients taking this drug for relief of narcolepsy also lost weight. As a result, amphetamine was soon being hailed as a virtual panacea for obesity. Unfortunately this enthusiastic claim, based, as it was, on uncontrolled observations, was not substantiated by controlled clinical trials. These revealed that while racemic amphetamine and its dextro rotatory isomer dexamphetamine in doses of 5–10 mg three times daily did lead to greater weight loss than a placebo, it was not as potent or effective as had been originally suggested. The mean daily weight loss of patients receiving these trials of amphetamines varied from 33–125 g depending on the trial, whereas the mean daily weight loss on placebo ranged from 13–85 g. These differences in daily weight loss between treatments are equivalent to 2–4 kg (4·4–8·8 lb) over a period of three months. It may be assumed that the increased weight loss which can be attributed to amphetamine medication is due to a reduced calorie intake, which in turn, as we have seen, is a consequence of the diminution in subjective hunger produced by the drug. Unfortunately within a matter of some six to twelve weeks tolerance develops and doses which have previously significantly reduced hunger will no longer do so.

As has already been discussed, amphetamine has a pronounced stimulating effect on the central nervous system, an effect which has led to its abuse by those of unstable personality seeking psychological arousal. Furthermore, prolonged administration of even relatively small doses (not more than 15 mg daily) can lead to psychological dependence, and overweight patients originally prescribed an amphetamine-containing preparation to help them keep to a reducing diet have found that when they are deprived of their tablets they become sluggish and depressed. Although such symptoms·last only a matter of a few days after stopping the drug, most patients find them sufficiently unpleasant to request, and in some cases demand, further supplies. Because of these effects the use of amphetamine in the treatment of obesity is no longer advisable.

In addition to central effects these compounds have some sympathomimetic activity which can lead to other side-effects such as dryness of the mouth. There is some risk of amphetamine causing a rise in blood pressure and tachycardia, both of which could be dangerous in anyone with a reduced cardiac reserve; also recent reports have been received of pulmonary hypertension following amphetamine administration. Such observations only add weight to the viewpoint that the disadvantages of amphetamine far outweigh any benefit it may possess.

2 *Phenmetrazine* (*Preludin*) Phenmetrazine was introduced as an anorectic in the hope that it would show fewer undesirable effects than amphetamine. Unfortunately this was found not to be the case; it shares all the disadvantages of the amphetamines and it too has been widely abused.

3 *Diethylpropion* (*Tenuate, Apisate*) While diethylpropion has an anorectic effect equal to that of amphetamine, clinically it does not appear to produce the same degree of central stimulation as amphetamine or phenmetrazine. Equally the risk of drug dependence seems to be less. Nevertheless, there is good experimental evidence to suggest that it can have a stimulant effect on the CNS as measured by CFF, and caution should therefore be applied when prescribing it.

Several controlled studies have revealed its efficacy in the treatment of obesity with daily weight losses of 20–80 g being directly attributable to the anorectic effect produced. It has shown to be the most effective when taken in doses of 50 mg one and one-half to two hours before meals. Equally effective clinically is the long-acting preparation (Tenuate dospan) which contains 75 mg diethylpropion in a slow release form.

4 *Phentermine (Duromine) and Chlorphentermine (Lucofen)* The first of these compounds when prescribed intermittently (30 mg daily) over a period of thirty-six weeks was found to be as effective, in terms of weight loss, as continuous administration, and more effective than placebo.

Chlorphentermine too is significantly more effective (in doses of 75 mg daily) than placebo in helping obese patients lose weight; patients lose some 50–120 g a day more with an active medication than with placebo. It is reported to have appreciably less stimulant activity than amphetamine.

5 *Fenfluramine (Ponderax)* Clinically, fenfluramine (in doses from 40–120 mg daily) is an effective adjunct to weight reduction regimes, being associated with weight losses similar to those of the other compounds previously discussed. Its main distinction from those compounds is its complete lack of any stimulant properties; if anything, it has a mild sedative action which is particularly useful in the treatment of those obese patients who also show signs of anxiety. Unfortunately it too has drawbacks, being prone to produce gastrointestinal side-effects, particularly diarrhoea, and acute confusional states following fenfluramine administration have been observed, particularly among patients who were receiving monoamine oxidase inhibitors at the same time.

6 *Biguanide compounds—Metformin (Glucophage) and phenformin (Dibotin)* While these compounds certainly assist obese diabetics in losing weight, their place in the treatment of uncomplicated obesity is still uncertain. At present their use should be restricted to those obese patients who are also suffering from diabetes mellitus, or who are thought to be pre-diabetic; for these patients the biguanides would appear to be the treatment of choice. The recommended doses are: metformin 0·5–1·0 g or phenformin 25–50 mg, three times daily.

7 *Bulk agents—Methylcellulose (Cellevac, Cellucon)* As there is no reliable clinical or experimental evidence to substantiate the claim that methylcellulose reduces hunger or food intake, preparations containing methylcellulose have little place in the treatment of obesity.

8 *General recommendations* It cannot be stressed too strongly or too often that successful weight reduction can only result from

reducing intake of calories to a level below that expended. All the preparations discussed above can therefore only be considered as possible adjuncts to a sensible dietary programme and never as complete treatments in themselves.

Furthermore, if an appetite-suppressant drug is used it should be prescribed intermittently and not continuously; patients should be on the drug for one or two months at the most, spending a similar period without medication before it is prescribed again. With these provisos, diethylpropion, phentermine or chlorphentermine would appear the most suitable anorectic compounds for depressed, lethargic, obese patients, while fenfluramine is probably better for the anxious, overactive patient. Obese diabetics should benefit most from one of the biguanide compounds.

Anorexia nervosa (Psychogenic malnutrition)

Anorexia nervosa is a condition in which severe malnutrition occurs as a result of a deliberate attempt by the patient to lose weight, usually because of a pathological fear of being fat. This characteristically takes the form of drastic reduction in calorie intake, although self-induced vomiting or frequent purgation may also be practised.

Anorexia nervosa most often begins during adolescence or in early adult life, affecting females far more frequently than males. In girls, amenorrhoea supervenes sooner or later. Despite the name of the condition, appetite is preserved in many cases. The emaciation produced, although alarming, is completely reversible by dietary measures.

The place of drugs in this condition, if any, is to assist the patient to keep to the diet and thereby gain weight. Apart from general sedation which may be required in the case of a particularly uncooperative patient, certain drugs are considered by some to have a particular value in helping patients to gain weight; these are chlorpromazine and insulin.

1 *Chlorpromazine* (*Largactil*) Chlorpromazine and to a lesser degree other phenothiazine derivatives frequently increase appetite and produce weight gain in psychiatric patients requiring to take them over long periods. In addition they have a marked sedative effect. It is just this combination of hunger stimulation and sedation which is particularly suitable for anorexia nervosa.

In many patients, however, no such medication is required as they readily settle in hospital and regain their appetite spontaneously, if they ever lose it. For those who do not respond to such relatively simple measures, chlorpromazine can usefully be prescribed in doses from 100 mg three times daily, increasing to the level of tolerance. Care must be taken to avoid over-sedation and the occurrence of parkinsonian symptoms will require appropriate anti-parkinsonian medication, together with a reduction in dosage of chlorpromazine.

A complication observed in some 10 per cent of the patients receiving chlorpromazine for anorexia nervosa is grand mal epilepsy, probably associated with fluid shifts.

2 *Insulin* As we have seen, subcutaneous injection of insulin leads to an increase in hunger some thirty minutes later. It is therefore not surprising that insulin has long been used to encourage patients with anorexia nervosa to eat, but obviously this measure will only be of value in those patients who are truly anorectic. The usual practice is to begin by injecting 10 units of soluble insulin one hour after breakfast. The dosage is then increased each day until sweating and slight drowsiness is produced; when these effects are observed a meal is offered to the patient, which, if eaten, will counter them. In general 40–60 units prove sufficient for the purpose. Patients receiving this treatment must be closely observed for several hours after the injection and a 20-ml-syringe containing a solution of glucose suitable for intravenous administration must be kept readily available in case sudden profound hypoglycaemia occurs.

3 *Cyproheptadine* (Periactin) A controlled trial of cyproheptadine in anorexia nervosa has revealed that it is probably of some benefit in the treatment of anorexia nervosa, particularly where this is undertaken under out-patient conditions.

Suggestions for further reading

ANAND, B. K., 'Nervous regulation of food intake', *Physiological Reviews*, Vol. 41, p. 677, 1961.

BAIRD, I. M., and HOWARD, A. N., *Obesity, Medical and Scientific Aspects*, E. S. Livingstone, Edinburgh, 1969.

BLISS, E. L., and BRANCH, C. H. H., *Anorexia Nervosa: Its History, Psychology and Biology*, Hoeber, New York, 1960.

CRADDOCK, D., *Obesity and its Management*, E. S. Livingstone, Edinburgh, 1969.

DALLY, P., *Anorexia Nervosa*, Heinemann Medical Books, London, 1969.

KENNEDY, G., 'Food intake, energy, balance and growth', *British Medical Bulletin*, Vol. 22, p. 216, 1966.

SILVERSTONE, J. T., and STUNKARD, A. J., 'The anorectic effect of dexamphetamine sulphate', *British Journal of Pharmacology and Chemotherapy*, Vol. 33, p. 513, 1968.

TEITELBAUM, P., 'Appetite', *Proceedings of the American Philosophic Society*, Vol. 108, p. 464, 1964.

Psychophysiology of pain

Pain is more than a modality of sensation like vision, hearing or touch; it is the integrated behavioural response of an individual to a noxious stimulus, either real or imagined. The experience of pain response depends not only on the intensity of the stimulus, but also on its central interpretation. As Merskey puts it 'pain is a psychological experience of events, occurring within the patient's own body, which is always unpleasant and associated with the impression of damage to the tissues'. Pain is by no means restricted to patients with organic disease; on the contrary a considerable proportion (about 60 per cent) of patients subsequently labelled 'psychiatric' present with symptoms of pain to their general practitioners. In general medical clinics of hospitals some 40 per cent of the patients, in whom the condition is considered to be primarily a psychiatric one, complain of pain. Such non-organic pain is commonly located in the head or trunk and has an arbitrary time course, unrelated to such events as eating, posture or exercise.

Even obviously organically determined pain can be greatly affected by psychological factors. For instance in 1943 Beecher noted at Anzio that soldiers with severe war wounds complained more about clumsy venepunctures than of their lacerations. Furthermore, their analgesic requirements were often small when compared with those for more trivial injuries away from the immediate stress of battle. Another example of the close relationship between the appreciation of pain and other psychological functions is provided in the case of neuroleptic analgesia; in this technique, potent narcotic and tranquillising drugs produce changes in a patient's interpretation of stimuli, so that major surgical procedures may be carried out in the conscious state without a painful response, even though local or general anaesthetic agents have not been given.

Such observations cast serious doubt on the *specificity theory* of pain sensation which was accepted for more than a century by eminent neurologists, such as Charles Bell, Weber, Brown-Sequard and von Frey. According to this theory pain is a specific modality like vision and hearing, and possesses its own peripheral and central apparatus. The peripheral component was thought to involve the free nerve endings in the dermis. Sir Henry Head distinguished between two types of pain, one sharp (epicritic) and the other dull (protopathic), and later investigators suggested that these were mediated by nerve fibres of different size and conduction velocities. There were important drawbacks to this theory, however, and a *pattern theory* was put forward by Goldschneider, in which he postulated that the appreciation of pain depended upon both the stimulus intensity and on central summation of the afferent impulses. These two viewpoints have been linked by Melzack and Wall, into the *gate-control theory*.

Gate-control theory of pain

It is known that stimulation of the skin evokes nerve impulses that are transmitted to three systems of nerves in the spinal cord:

(i) the cells of the substantia gelatinosa in the dorsal horn of the cord
(ii) the fibres in the dorsal column that run upwards towards the brain
(iii) the first central transmission cells (T) in the dorsal horn.

Melzack and Wall proposed that the cells of the substantia gelatinosa function as a 'gate' which regulates transmission from the peripheral fibres from the skin to the T cells. The patterns of activity in the ascending neurones of the dorsal column regulate central brain processes which in turn influence the 'gate-control' activity of the cells of the substantia gelatinosa through descending fibres. Finally, the T cells activate the neural mechanisms responsible for response and perception. In other words, the cells of the substantia gelatinosa regulate the level of stimulation by impulses from the periphery of the T cells (which are the first stage of the central pain response and perception system). The amount of stimulation which these 'gate' cells permit is dependent on inhibitory and excitatory activity in large and small fibres respectively from the periphery, and on inhibition and excitation through descending pathways from the brain (see Figure 2).

This theory not only reconciles the specificity and pattern theories of pain perception, but is also consistent with other phenomena concerned with pain. For example, the intense pain associated with some forms of peripheral neuropathy, such as that due to diabetes or alcoholism, may be explained by a reduction in the normal inhibition of input by the gate-control system, because of selective large fibre destruction in these conditions.

It is probable that gating and selection of sensory information takes place at many levels of the central nervous system and that centrally acting drugs may influence this activity at various levels, so producing varying degrees and types of alteration in pain perception and response.

Nature of nociceptors

Although pain may be produced by many different forms of tissue injury, it is possible that the actual stimulus common to all is chemical. A wide variety of substances produce pain when applied to exposed dermis; these include acids, alkaloids, hypo- and hypertonic solutions, histamine, 5-hydroxytryptamine, acetylcholine and several polypeptides including bradykinin, angiotensin and vasopressin. It is likely that physical forms of injury produce their painful effects by releasing similar substances in the tissues, and it is probable that 'pain receptor' itself is chemical in nature. The term 'chemoceptor' has been coined to apply to such a receptor, which is unlikely to have a specific chemical structure, as there is such a large variety of pain-producing agents. Furthermore, it is possible that other compounds, by attaching themselves to chemoceptors, might prevent pain-producing substances from approaching the receptors sufficiently closely for binding, thus preventing the painful response. There is experimental evidence to suggest that the antipyretic analgesics act in this way.

Pharmacology of analgesic drugs

Peripheral action

Experiments with bradykinin-induced pain in animals and man indicate that antipyretic-analgesic drugs such as aspirin act, in part at least, by blocking the chemoceptors for pain. It is probable that paracetamol and phenacetin have a similar action. In keeping with this is the relative lack of central actions of these drugs when compared with the narcotic analgesics.

Central action

The most important group of centrally acting analgesic drugs are the narcotic compounds derived from the opium alkaloids, or structurally related to them. These include the potent analgesics morphine and diamorphine, and the weaker dihydrocodeine and codeine. The actual site and mode of action of these compounds is not known for certain, although it is probable that thalamic centres are particularly involved. However, they all possess other central effects, including sedation and respiratory depression. The narcotic antagonist compounds pentazocine and cyclazocine, which antagonise the sedation and respiratory depressant activity of the narcotic analgesics, also possess some analgesic activity which is significantly less than that of the narcotic analgesics, but may, nevertheless, be of therapeutic value. Pentazocine, in particular, has become widely used, but although its dependence-producing properties are much lower than morphine, dependence to it has been described in a few cases, and central effects of dysphoria and hallucinations are not uncommon.

The narcotic analgesic drugs can all produce severe disturbances of sensation, leading at times to hallucinations, if given in large doses. Bradley has suggested that these analgesic and hallucinogenic actions are closely inter-related in their basic pharmacological mechanism, analgesia being a form of disturbance of sensory function similar to that which occurs in drug-induced hallucinations. In favour of this notion is the finding that the potent hallucinogen lysergic acid diethylamide (LSD) has been shown to interfere with the flow of sensory information to the cerebral cortex in animals.

Although not of therapeutic analgesic importance when used alone, some other centrally acting drugs can be shown to raise the pain threshold in animals and man. Among these are amphetamine, a central stimulant drug, and chlorpromazine, a central depressant compound. Once again, the mechanism of their analgesic effects is unknown.

Interactions of analgesic drugs

The effects of the narcotic analgesic drugs may be increased by simultaneous administration of other drugs, particularly those of the neuroleptic group such as phenothiazines and butyrophenones. These compounds are thought to act primarily by modifying entry of information into the reticular formation of the brain stem, and it is probable that their interaction with analgesic compounds is dependent on this. At the same time they help to reduce anxiety associated with the presence of severe pain, especially when this is due to malignancy.

Neuroleptanalgesia is a term given to the state of analgesia obtained by the combination of a neuroleptic agent and an analgesic of short duration. The neuroleptics most commonly used for this purpose are phenothiazines or phenothiazine derivatives, such as chlorprothixine, and butyrophenones such as droperidol. The analgesics are essentially of the morphine type: moramide, phenoperidine and phentanyl. The two types of drugs are usually given by continuous intravenous infusion. Although the patient so treated has a tendency to sleep, he need not do so, but is not particularly provoked by traumatic procedures such as surgical operation, which would normally be intolerably painful to him, thus producing a clinical state of shock. An essential part of the phenomenon is the protection of the patient against the autonomic effects of pain by selectively blocking the various cellular, autonomic and endocrine mechanisms normally active during stress. The patient is usually conscious, but not capable of prolonged attention. The corneal reflex is present, and the skin is pink, warm and dry; there is muscular hypotension and relaxation, while the respiratory rate is low and the volume increased; arterial pressure and heart rate is reduced, but tissue perfusion remains satisfactory as cardiac output increases with an associated diuresis. Body temperature usually falls, particularly when chlorprothixine is used. After recovery the patient is calm, without nausea or vomiting and remains amnesic for the procedure.

Neuroleptanalgesia emphasises the importance of central nervous factors in mediating the normal pain responses to noxious stimuli, and the way in which modification of central function may influence the nature of these responses, both physiological and autonomic.

Clinical aspects

The choice of analgesic drug for a particular patient depends on several factors:

1 *The nature of the pain-producing pathology* When pain is associated with malignancy or myocardial infarction, sedation, as well as analgesia, is required. In such circumstances the narcotic analgesic compounds with their central sedating action are to be preferred to peripherally acting compounds. Such considerations also occur frequently after surgical procedures. In the case of non-malignant conditions, however, the number of doses should be limited to the minimum necessary to relieve pain, in order to reduce the risk of development of dependence. Pain associated with inflammatory conditions, particularly the musculoskeletal system, is better treated with antipyretic-analgesic compounds having a peripheral action.

2 *The severity of the pain* It is a therapeutic maxim that the mildest analgesic compound should be used which produces adequate pain relief. When a peripherally acting compound is required, therefore, paracetamol and aspirin should be used before the more potent, but potentially more dangerous, compounds such as phenylbutazone (Butazolidin) and indomethacin (Indocid). Similarly, codeine and dihydrocodeine have markedly less central depressant, hallucinogenic and dependence-producing activity than the more potent compounds such as pethidine, morphine and diamorphine. Pentazocine (Fortral), a narcotic antagonist, is a weaker analgesic than morphine, but its dependence-producing properties are also less.

If a potent narcotic analgesic drug is used for only slight pain, its side-effects may more than outweigh its therapeutic advantages. In controlled clinical trials in post-operative pain, pethidine 100 mg has been found to be not significantly different from placebo when all the patients were considered overall, but if they were subdivided according to initial severity of their pain, then the drug was found to be very effective in those with severe pain, but of no value in those with only slight pain. Conversely, aspirin 600 mg was of no demonstrable value in the patient population taken overall, but was very effective in the patients with mild pain, and of little or no value in those with severe pain. This difference probably reflects the greater weight patients attach to side-effects if their pain is only slight, or if the analgesic drug is producing inadequate pain relief.

The severity of pain after any operative procedure varies greatly from patient to patient, and the practice of routine prescription of regular potent narcotic analgesic drugs for all patients after surgical operations should be discouraged. Treatment should only be prescribed after full consideration of individual requirements, even though this may take up more of the doctor's time.

3 *Other treatment which the patient is receiving* The analgesic activity of the narcotic drugs, in particular, is increased by neuroleptic drugs of the phenothiazine and butyrophenone type. For this reason smaller doses than normal of the analgesic drug may be required in patients already receiving one of the neuroleptics. Similarly, where a patient is becoming tolerant to the analgesic activity of a drug, its effectiveness may be increased by the addition of a neuroleptic to the treatment regime. This has the added advantage of reducing still further any anxiety component which may be present.

Monoamine oxidase inhibitors (see chapter 6) can also interact with narcotic analgesics, particularly pethidine, to produce profound depression of central nervous function. Various disturbances may occur such as excitation, rigidity, coma, changes in blood pressure, shock and hyperpyrexia. The basic biochemical mechanism of this interaction and its manifestations is uncertain. It is of great importance that patients receiving treatment with MAO inhibitors and who require surgical procedures should only be given pethidine with considerable caution.

4 *The psychology of the patient* The evaluation of drugs in the relief of pain is difficult, and some well controlled trials have failed to show that drugs as potent as morphine are much superior to the weaker compounds, or even a placebo (see chapter 4).

When there are grounds for feeling that a patient may be abnormally suggestible, then it may be justified to present a very weak or even inactive preparation as a preliminary therapeutic trial. If he or she responds, then the risks of serious side-effects are proportionally lower than with an active drug, even though placebo-induced side-effects are frequently described by such patients.

As we have seen, pain may be largely, if not entirely, psycho-

logically determined in many cases. Merskey and Spear have classified the situations in which this can occur as follows: (i) psychological factors (particularly anxiety or depression) which initiate
or exacerbate local physical disturbances (ii) hysterical conversion
syndromes (iii) delusions or hallucinations occurring as part of a
major psychiatric illness, either affective or schizophrenic.

In the first group where anxiety exacerbates the situation, an
anxiolytic sedative (see chapter 7), or an antidepressant (see chapter
6), where the pain is a feature of an underlying depressive illness,
will often by themselves be sufficient to relieve the pain. Muscular
pains of the tension type are common in anxiety states and pain is a
frequent feature of depressive illness. In the latter condition the
pain may be a recurrence of past organically determined pain, or
it may represent a preoccupation with bodily sensations which are
normally well tolerated when the patient is well.

Pain occurring as a manifestation of conversion hysteria requires specialist psychiatric treatment. Anxiolytic sedatives and
antidepressants are unlikely to help, while the narcotic analgesics
should not be given, because of the serious risk of producing drug
dependency (Eugene O'Neill's play, *A Long Day's Journey into
Night* provides a grim example of this).

Figure 2 *Diagram to illustrate role of substantia gelatinosa in acting
as a gate-control system in regulating input of sensory information into
the central nervous pathways concerned with the perception of, and
response to, pain*

If pain occurs as a feature of either a delusion or a hallucinatory experience the appropriate action is treatment of the psychosis (see chapter 5 for treatment of schizophrenia and chapter 6 for treatment of affective disorders).

Suggestion for further reading

MERSKY, H., and SPEAR, F. G., *Pain, Psychological and Psychiatric Aspects*, Ballière, Tindall & Cassell, London, 1967.

Child psychiatry 14

In general, drug treatment has but a limited place in child psychiatry. The majority of cases presenting to the child psychiatrist require social and psychotherapeutic support rather than pharmacological intervention. Nevertheless, there are certain syndromes which do benefit from psychotropic drugs; these include behaviour disturbance in brain-damaged or epileptic children, school refusal, nocturnal enuresis, some cases of stammering and certain patients with motor tics. Those very rare cases of true schizophrenia which occur during the later stages of childhood respond to neuroleptic drugs in a similar fashion to adults (see chapter 5).

Behaviour disturbance in brain-damaged children

It is now generally recognised that psychiatric disorder is common among children showing evidence of brain damage, the most frequent abnormality being antisocial behaviour. Other syndromes thought to be a reflection of underlying cerebral pathology include the hyperkinetic syndrome, aggressive outbursts and autistic behaviour. Many brain-damaged children also suffer from epilepsy and, where this occurs, adequate control of epileptic attacks will often improve the situation considerably. Control may be achieved by phenytoin (Epanutin) 60–200 mg daily, primidone (Mysoline) 100–500 mg daily, carbamazepine (Tegretol) 100–500 mg daily, sulthiame (Ospolot) 60–300 mg daily. In addition the latter compound has been reported to improve behaviour in disturbed mentally handicapped patients who are not epileptic. As phenobarbitone tends to exacerbate behaviour disorders it should be avoided where possible in the management of epileptic children who manifest disturbed behaviour.

In addition to epilepsy there may be other associated neurological abnormalities which further complicate the life of the brain-damaged child. Thus the management of behaviour disturbance in children with brain damage encompasses rather more than just the prescription of an appropriate drug; a comprehensive social, psychological and physical approach is required.

Hyperkinetic syndrome

The hyperkinetic syndrome (which is thought to be a reflection of underlying brain damage) is characterised by extreme restlessness and distractability, usually coming on between the ages of two and five. There may or may not be frank neurological signs. Epilepsy, which complicates the picture in almost half the cases, should be controlled with a suitable anticonvulsant (see above).

Symptomatic benefit can often be obtained with a neuroleptic drug (see chapter 5), the most widely used being chlorpromazine (Largactil, Thorazine) 10–25 mg three times daily. Alternatively, haloperidol (Serenace, Haldol) can be administered unobtrusively as drops added to food in a dose of 0·05 mg/kg per day.

Paradoxically, dexamphetamine (Dexedrine), which has an arousing effect in adults, has a calmative effect on hyperkinetic activity in children; an appropriate dose is 5–10 mg daily; this may be increased to a maximum of 40 mg. Methylphenidate (Ritalin) 10–60 mg daily is an equally effective alternative. These drugs do however have some serious potential disadvantages. First, the side-effects of insomnia, tachycardia and anorexia may prove troublesome, although the insomnia can be reduced by giving the drug early in the day. Second, and of even greater potential danger, is the definite risk of producing drug dependence in later years. It has been reported that the incidence of drug abuse is higher among those children with the hyperkinetic syndrome who have received amphetamine in the past. Thus administration of these drugs should be strictly limited to those children with unequivocal symptoms and signs of the condition. Even among these there is a very good chance that considerable improvement will occur by adolescence. It is therefore recommended that when amphetamines are prescribed, they should be stopped from time to time to see if they are still required.

Aggressive outbursts

The behaviour of brain-damaged children may be punctuated by short-lived outbursts of extreme aggression and destructiveness.

These episodic symptoms can be ameliorated by neuroleptic drugs of the phenothiazine type (e.g. chlorpromazine) or the butyrophenone type (e.g. haloperidol), given in the same doses as for the hyperkinetic syndrome (see above). A relatively uncommon condition, Gilles de la Tourette's syndrome, in which an attack of severe motor tics is accompanied by a stream of obscenities, is said to respond best to haloperidol.

School refusal and panic attacks

The extreme reluctance to go to school displayed by some children is not so much a phobia of school itself, but rather a fear of leaving the security of the home. It must be distinguished from other causes of non-attendance at school, in particular truancy, which is a reflection of an antisocial attitude rather than of anxiety.

Although the majority of school refusers can be handled successfully without recourse to drugs, in some cases, particularly when there have been panic attacks, an anxiolytic sedative of the benzodiazepine type (see chapter 7) can reduce anxiety sufficiently to allow the child to contemplate going back to school. Chlordiazepoxide (Librium) 5–10 mg two or three times daily and diazepam (Valium) 2–5 mg three times daily are both suitable for this purpose.

Nocturnal enuresis

Nocturnal enuresis, or bedwetting at night, can be considered abnormal if it persists after the age of five. It is now generally believed to be the result of delayed maturation, rather than secondary to emotional problems. In favour of this view is the observation that almost all enuretic children become completely dry at night by the time they leave school. As an approximation, some 15 per cent of children aged five frequently wet the bed at night; this figure falls to 5 per cent among 10-year-olds, and to 1 per cent by the age of 15. Rarely, nocturnal enuresis is a symptom of structural abnormality of the urinary tract, but in those cases there is usually incontinence by day as well as by night.

If physical examination and urinalysis fail to reveal any abnormality, and the sole symptom is bedwetting, the condition is almost certainly primary nocturnal enuresis, and further investigation is rarely called for.

Drug treatment appears to help some children affected by this problem, although as yet no drug has been nearly as effective as conditioning treatment (using a bell and pad apparatus). Nevertheless, as drugs are so much easier to administer they are usually worth a limited trial in the first instance.

Three groups of compounds have been used: anticholinergic drugs, stimulants and tricyclic antidepressants.

Anticholinergic drugs

These act by blocking the parasympathetic innervation to the bladder. By decreasing bladder irritability and increasing urethral resistance and bladder capacity they delay bladder emptying. A wide variety of preparations have been tried, including the belladonna alkaloids, and synthetic compounds such as methantheline (Banthine) 15 mg at night, propantheline (Pro-Banthine) 15 mg at night, and isopropamide (Tyrimide) 5 mg at night. The results of treatment with these anticholinergic drugs have been generally disappointing.

Sympathomimetic compounds

Substances such as dexamphetamine sulphate (Dexedrine), methylamphetamine (Methedrine) 5–10 mg and ephedrine 60 mg given before retiring have a dual action which would appear to be of potential benefit to enuretic subjects. They act centrally to raise cerebral arousal and should thereby lessen the depth of sleep, allowing the subject to awaken more easily when his bladder fills. They also act on the sympathetic innervation to the bladder, causing contraction of the vesical sphincter. Whatever their theoretical advantages, these drugs are of only occasional benefit in practice, and double-blind trials have not revealed any clear-cut superiority over placebo.

Tricyclic antidepressant compounds

Probably by virtue of their associated anticholinergic effects together with their known potentiation of adrenergic activity (see chapter 2), tricyclic antidepressant drugs, such as imipramine (Tofranil), amitriptyline (Tryptizol, Elavil) and nortriptyline (Aventyl), in a dose of 25–50 mg at night, have been shown to be of greater effectiveness than placebo in reducing the frequency of bedwetting. Although this is of some benefit, they only achieve the complete remission which most patients (and their parents) seek in 20 per cent of cases. Nevertheless, treatment with one of these preparations would seem to be a reasonable first step in management. If successful within three or four weeks then medication should be continued for at least another month before being cautiously reduced over the ensuing few months. Relapse during this time calls for raising the dose to the level at which a favourable response had been achieved.

If tricyclic drugs in adequate dosage fail to produce an adequate improvement within four weeks there is little point in persevering with this line of treatment, particularly as cases of tricyclic poisoning are increasing among children.

Stuttering (Stammering)

Frequent interruption of the free flow of speech, severe enough to interfere with communication, which is made worse by conscious efforts to overcome it, characterises the condition of stuttering. While this may occur to some degree in up to 3 per cent of children, only 1 per cent become persistent stutterers. As far as drug treatment is concerned, haloperidol 0·75–1·5 mg three times a day (when combined with speech therapy) has been shown to be better than a placebo given under the same conditions. Behavioural techniques which train the child to speak in a strict rhythm (by using a metronome) are also of value. Combinations of drugs with such behaviour therapy have yet to be evaluated.

Tics

Tics may be defined as brief, jerky involuntary movements, which occur particularly in the muscles around the eyes and lower part of the face. They are relatively common, being present in up to 5 per cent of all children at some time; the time they are most likely to occur is between the ages of five and ten. Tics are usually exacerbated by emotional distress, and are more frequently found in boys. Drugs of the anxiolytic sedative type such as the benzodiazepines (e.g. chlordiazepoxide 5–10 mg or diazepam 2–5 mg three times daily) may help reduce the emotional component of the condition and thereby reduce the frequency of the tics. Haloperidol 0·5–1·5 mg three times daily has also been found to be of benefit, although the larger dose may lead to extrapyramidal effects.

Suggestions for further reading

BARKER, P., *Basic Child Psychiatry*, Staples Press, London, 1971.

BLACKWELL, B., and CURRAN, J., 'The psychopharmacology of nocturnal enuresis', *Little Club Clinics in Development Medicine*, 1973.

FISH, B., 'Drug use in psychiatric disorders of children', *American Journal of Psychiatry*, Vol. 124, pp. 31–6, 1968.

VAN PRAAG, H. M., 'Psychotropic drugs in child psychiatry', *International Pharmacopsychiatry*, Vol. 3, pp. 137–54, 1969.

YOUNG, G., 'The problem of enuresis', *British Journal of Hospital Medicine*, Vol. 2, pp. 628–32, 1969.

Appendix

Notes on the management of overdosage of centrally acting drugs

Self-poisoning with centrally acting drugs, particularly barbiturates and other hypnotics, is the commonest method of suicide in the United Kingdom. There are certain general principles which apply to the treatment of such self-poisoning, irrespective of the actual substance ingested.

Maintenance of respiration

Respiratory depression occurs with many centrally acting drugs, particularly the barbiturates and other hyponotics. In addition, there may be airway obstruction due to inhalation of vomitus or to excessive mucous production. It is, therefore, of the utmost importance to ensure a clear airway, if necessary by insertion of a cuffed endotracheal tube or even by tracheostomy. If the patient is cyanosed, or in fact if there is any suspicion of inadequate ventilation, oxygen should be administered in high concentration, and intermittent positive pressure respiration considered. If facilities are available the minute volume may be measured with a Wright's spirometer and arterial blood gas analysis carried out at regular intervals. There is no place for the use of analeptic drugs in overdosage with psychotropic drugs. They have a narrow therapeutic ratio and readily produce epileptiform convulsions and cardiac dysrhythmias.

Maintenance of cardiovascular function

Depression of the vasomotor and cardiac centres may occur with many centrally acting drugs. In addition, prolonged vomiting or excessive sweating can cause marked fluid depletion and lead to a state of hypotension and shock. This results in increased sympathetic activity with peripheral vasoconstriction and shunting of blood from skin and splanchnic areas to maintain adequate coronary and cerebral perfusion. Inadequate perfusion of the lungs may lead to metabolic acidosis.

The central venous pressure should be measured and if it is reduced, intravenous fluids should be infused cautiously to increase the circulating volume and cardiac output. However, if there is any suggestion of incipient renal failure with acute tubular necrosis (see below) infusion should be delayed; equally it must be discontinued if signs of fluid excess appear. The use of vasoconstrictor agents such as noradrenaline or metaraminol is controversial. On theoretical grounds it is unlikely to be of much value because sympathetic tone is already high in most shocked patients and the administration of alpha-receptor stimulating drugs may well further decrease tissue perfusion in organs such as the gut and kidney. If rehydration fails to raise the blood pressure to acceptable levels, intravenous hydrocortisone 100 mg should be given and repeated at regular intervals as necessary. Many psychotropic drugs produce cardiac dysrhythmias and cardiac monitoring should, therefore, be employed where possible during the recovery period in all patients.

Control of convulsions

Convulsions may occur in overdosage with central stimulant and antidepressant compounds, and also in phenothiazine and 'Mandrax' poisoning in which the epileptic seizure threshold is reduced. They can be controlled by intramuscular injection of phenobarbitone sodium 300 mg, phenytoin sodium 250 mg, diazepam 10 mgs or paraldehyde 10 ml, repeated as necessary. If severe respiratory depression occurs, mechanical ventilation should be used.

Reduction of absorption

When it is known that the drug concerned has been ingested within four hours of admission to hospital, it is reasonable to attempt to prevent further absorption by emptying the patient's stomach. If the patient is conscious it may be possible to induce emesis by pharyngeal stimulation or administration of strong salt solution. The alternative for the unconscious or semiconscious patient is gastric lavage, but this is a potentially dangerous procedure, and must be avoided if there is any suspicion that the patient may have taken corrosives or petroleum substances, and in patients known to have upper alimentary disease. After gastric lavage has been carried out, purgation may be induced by means of 50–100 ml of 70 per cent sorbitol solution given via the gastric tube, so emptying the small bowel of its contents of drug and preventing further absorption.

Increase in rate of drug elimination

1   *Diuresis*   In the absence of renal impairment, the patient's kidneys provide a better dialysing membrane than any artificial kidney for the

elimination of a drug. However, because renal impairment may have been present before the drug ingestion, or a state of profound hypotension might have induced acute tubular necrosis, the ability of the kidneys to excrete a fluid load should be assessed before attempting to force a diuresis. This may be done by administering intravenously a small volume of 10 or 20 per cent mannitol and observing the urinary output during the next few minutes. If there is a significant increase in urine output, it is reasonable to proceed with provoking a diuresis. If not, then intravenous infusion of fluids may precipitate left ventricular failure and pulmonary oedema; in that case other methods of drug elimination must be considered.

When a diuresis is to be produced, two factors must be considered, namely its volume and the urinary pH. The relative importance of these factors differs according to the drug under consideration. When the reabsorption of the drug across the renal tubular membrane from the lumen of the tubule into the blood stream is not markedly pH dependent, then the only way to modify the rate of excretion is to increase the volume or urine and hence the rate at which it passes through the tubule. This minimises the time during which reabsorption of the drug may occur.

In the case of weak acids, such as salicyclic acid, acetylsalicylic acid, and phenobarbitone, and weak bases such as pethidine, morphine, chlorpromazine, amphetamine, ephedrine, the tricyclic antidepressants and tranylcypromine, alteration of the urinary pH may markedly influence the rate of excretion. The excretion of weakly acidic drugs is increased if the urine is made alkaline, usually by intravenous administration of 1/6 molar lactate solution. Conversely excretion of drugs which are weakly basic is increased if the urine is made more acid by oral or intravenous administration of ammonium chloride.

The intravenous administration of sufficient volumes of fluid, either dextrose or saline, may be enough to provoke and maintain an adequate diuresis, but it is common practice to use a diuretic agent as well, either an osmotic diuretic such as intravenous mannitol (for example 100 ml of 10 per cent mannitol diluted in 500 ml normal saline in one hour), or a diuretic which blocks sodium reabsorption such as frusemide 40–60 mg.

2 *Dialysis* Peritoneal or haemodialysis should be considered in order to increase the rate of elimination of a drug when blood levels are very high and the clinical condition is poor, or where renal insufficiency precludes the use of forced diuresis.

Care of the unconscious patient

Routine care of the unconscious patient should be scrupulously observed, with particular reference to the skin, with: two-hourly turning and use of a ripple bed if the patient remains unconscious for more than twelve hours; the bladder, with catheterisation under strict aseptic conditions; the bowels, with attention paid to evacuation; and hygiene of the mouth, nose and eyes. The nutritional state must also be observed, with institution of parenteral feeding if necessary.

Psychiatric assessment and treatment

During the recovery phase, the patient may become agitated, distressed or even violent, and may require sedation. If suicidal intent was originally suspected a full psychiatric assessment should be carried out after recovery.

Specific measures

In certain cases of poisoning with centrally acting drugs, additional specific measures may be indicated: narcotic antagonists, such as nalorphine, may be used in patients poisoned with morphine, heroin or pethidine, in order to reduce respiratory depression. However, an acute abstinence syndrome may be precipitated if physical dependence has developed on the narcotic drug.

Over-dosage of monoamine oxidase inhibitors may be associated with hyperpyrexia, for which chlorpromazine is the treatment of choice. If marked hypertension is present, this should be treated with an alpha-adrenergic receptor-blocking drug, such as phentolamine or thymoxamine.

Subject index

Index of drug names

Proprietary brand-names are printed in small capitals.